I0151801

WOMAN 2 WOMAN

Life Lessons Learned on the Journey
to Marriage, Motherhood, Entrepreneurship,
Divorce, Surviving Breast Cancer
and Finding New Love

Delphyne Lomax Taylor

Books by Anthony Parnell
Las Vegas, Nevada

AP
Anthony Parnell

www.Woman2Woman.Network

www.AnthonyParnell.com

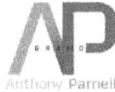

WOMAN 2 WOMAN
Life Lessons Learned on the Journey to Marriage, Motherhood,
Entrepreneurship, Divorce, Surviving Breast Cancer,
and Finding New Love

Copyright © 2020 by Delphyne Lomax Taylor

Books by Anthony Parnell
Las Vegas, Nevada

ISBN: 978-0-9644205-9-5

Library of Congress Control Number: 2020914475

Cover Design by Kire Thomas

WORDS OF GRATITUDE

Writing this book forced me to dig deep within to explore and uncover parts of myself that I didn't know existed or had buried many years ago. As a result, the process and journey of working on the manuscript evoked many emotions; thus, making the process that much more challenging. Now, having finally reached the finish line, I feel nothing but gratitude and a spirit of thanksgiving to so many family and friends who supported me along the way. They encouraged me to let go of my fears and to step out on faith in writing this book. More importantly, they helped me to see that I have a message to share with women all around the world: that, *Woman 2 Woman*, we need to have more honest and substantive conversations with one another.

A Special Thank You to

Sunserai Bell
Donald Lomax
Kathy Ragland
Falisha Riaye
Lisa Sales
Yvetta Young

for helping us get through our first edits.

NOTE: In the writing of this book, to protect the privacy of individuals, some names have been changed.

DEDICATION
TO FERN MCQUEEN

This book is dedicated to Fern McQueen. She is the reason that I am writing a book about my journey. When I was in the early stages of battling Breast Cancer, she gave me a journal to capture my thoughts day by day. She was also there during one of the most difficult times in my life, divorce. To my sister Fern, this is for You and all the other women in the world who I hope have the opportunity to read this book. Or, at the very least, they will be fortunate enough to experience the type of Friendship we had. Rest in Peace My Sister. Rest in Peace!

TABLE OF CONTENTS

INTRODUCTION

This book was inspired by my life experiences and those of countless women of all ages, races, and socioeconomic backgrounds. We all are susceptible to various forms of cancer. We all desire opportunities to grow personally and professionally. And, we all need a loving circle of support.

This book, then, seeks to engage readers in a conversation about such pertinent topics as: marriage; being a mother; divorce; finding new love; discovering one's life purpose; entrepreneurship; and, because I am a breast cancer survivor, increasing awareness of the importance of getting a yearly mammogram. This is essential because early detection is one of the key factors in surviving breast cancer.

The additional inspiration for writing this book was turning 60. For months leading up to my 60th birthday, I could feel an internal psychological and emotional shift taking place. Although I now am 62, over the last few years, I could feel myself coming to peace with the full realization and acceptance, that without my various life experiences, I would not be the person I am today. By no means am I suggesting that I am perfect. Rather, it is celebrating the fact that I no longer feel the self-imposed pressure to try to be perfect. I now am at a place in my life where I truly am at peace with myself, at peace with all of who I am. And, I am fully aware that this is a blessing, a gift in and of itself.

Turning 60 also spurred a feeling of not wanting to live my life with any regrets. At the top of my bucket list was always wanting to write a book about my life. Even though I've never considered myself a writer, I knew I had a powerful story to share with others about my journey, my struggles, and ultimately, my triumphs! In particular, I felt a calling to help and encourage other women who might be going through some of the same things I've gone through. This stems from the fact that I've always been a giving person, but, now, my thoughts of wisdom would become more tangible when put into a book, the written word.

Somehow, turning 60 for me was also symbolic of a new stage of personal growth. On many levels, I gradually was shedding years of baggage that I had been carrying around. As a result, I increasingly felt more empowered than ever. I was no longer willing or able to be a prisoner of my fear or even what for many years had really been procrastination.

Just as important as it is for me to share with you the internal growth that first had to take place in order for me to write this book, it's also important for me to share with you that the actual process of writing the book, in many ways, is just as significant as the process of gaining enough courage to write it.

As fate would have it, in December 2017, an email appeared in my box that read:

"Write or Publish Your Book in 6 Months or Less!!!"

Seeing this email blast resonated with something deep inside of me that had been there for quite some time. It was an intense desire to give birth to a book that could be shared with women who are going through or have gone through many of the same things that I had experienced in my life.

Without hesitating, I opened up the email and quickly realized it was not from someone unknown. Rather, it was from a family friend of more than 35 years, Anthony Parnell. Anthony was someone whom I had known since he was a teenager. In fact, my former husband and I had been his Sunday School teachers when he was in high school in our hometown of Akron, Ohio. So, even though we had lost contact for a number of years, having already known him made it that much easier to work through my fears. A few hours after reading his email, I decided to reach out to him about publishing my book.

After just one call, in less than thirty minutes, I knew he was the perfect person to help me write and publish my book. He not only was a published author himself. He was a gifted listener and synthesizer of my thoughts and emotions.

A few months later we started working on the book by scheduling and recording weekly calls. The approach we took was to first solely focus on getting all of my thoughts, feelings and recollections out and onto paper. This was to be accomplished without being critical of any of the content or ideas that we produced. We literally approached the initial stages of the creative process just as a painter or songwriter might do when starting from scratch in drawing a painting or writing a song. What resulted was a series of what I would call conversations. I say conversations because there was such a natural flow of back and forth dialogue that this is what it felt like to me.

Much to my surprise, being able to talk through my journey, chapter-by-chapter, became a very therapeutic process for me. This was much more than I ever anticipated gaining from the process of writing this book. Intermixed with this was the surprising realization, several weeks into the process, that I was feeling a level of comfort in sharing my story with a man rather than a woman. This extended from the most generic events of my life to the most intimate details that I had never shared with anyone.

I found this revelation to be very significant because one of the underlying themes of this book—in sharing several stories of pain and hurt that were inflicted intentionally and unintentionally by a number of men—is that through it all, I have not held on to bitterness. I have learned to trust and believe in the power of forgiveness to ensure that I don't become a prisoner of my past.

In the midst of my wounding, I never lost sense of the fact that the natural order of life is for us to grow as women and to reach our full potential. We, however, cannot do it in a vacuum outside of the context of men also playing an integral role in our lives. So, for a man to be the one to help me dig deep within myself, to tap into every word and emotion I had been longing to express for a number of years, is a representation of my life, and more importantly, my process of healing coming full circle.

Even more, the benefit for the reader, I believe, is that I was able to write a book that comes from a place of having a balanced perspective of the events of the past which have led me to this point in my life. And, at this point, I feel like a whole person despite the deep wounds I've endured. Subsequently, this book has evolved beyond being a book that is just about my experiences as a woman. It is a book for men as well. This is because it speaks to everyone's need for inspiration and life lessons along our journey that will help us heal, grow, reach our full potential and hopefully be empowered to manifest our deepest desires.

For many years, I had wanted to write a book about my life experiences but had never taken one step in that direction. So, now, to finally be able to see this dream come to light, for me, is a major accomplishment. Just the fact of knowing that I achieved a long unfulfilled major goal of publishing a book has given me such joy and a wonderful feeling inside. The icing on the cake is knowing that I have encouraged and inspired readers to make changes, bold changes in their lives for the better.

On a final note, spirituality is another powerful life force that I would like to mention and hopefully encourage more women to tap into. When I say spirituality, I am not speaking in a religious sense. I am speaking in a broader sense with regards to living our lives in a way that we live with purpose and we live with a greater sense of expectancy that blessings will constantly come our way; that the more we remove feelings of guilt and self-sabotaging thoughts and behavior, the more we find ourselves at the right place at the right time, and the more the right people appear in our lives to take us to another level.

When, I for example, was working on the final edits to this book, the book title *Woman 2 Woman*, caught my attention in a different way. More specifically, I zeroed in on the number 2. That's when it suddenly hit me that there must be special meaning to the number 2. When I did a Google search, look at what I discovered:

> In numerology, **2** represents partnerships, relationships, and harmony (balance). If your **Life Path number** is 2, you are a seeker after peace and harmony, with a fantastic sensitivity to other people and a desire to build the strongest relationships possible. (Source: trustedpsychicmediums.com)

> According to the **Bible**, the **number 2** is Eve's **number**; It is a symbol of union, which can be seen in different examples. We have the union between the church and Christ, as well as the union between a man and a woman in a marriage. (Source: angelnumbersmeaning.com)

So, in closing, may this book inspire you to live in love, harmony and partnerships that nurture you while holding you accountable and helping you reach your full potential. This includes the partnerships we have with one another as women, *Woman 2 Woman*.

Embrace the journey,

Delphyne Lomax Taylor

CHAPTER 1
AKRON, OHIO

Where someone is born can say a lot about them. If you're born in a tropical climate, the East Coast, the West Coast, and so on.

So, what does it mean that I was born in Akron, Ohio? The Rubber Capital of the world. The home of the Soap Box Derby. The city where Alcoholics Anonymous (AA) was founded by Bill Wilson and Bob Smith. During the 50s and 60s, not only was Akron filled with a rich history and a strong sense of community, there was a plethora of jobs. This was the impetus for many African-Americans migrating from the South.

In fact, there was a good twenty to fifty-year run where you had your pick of the litter in deciding which company to work for. You had companies like Firestone, Goodyear and Goodrich all in the same city. Because of this abundance of well-paying jobs which continued into the 70s and 80s, many of my classmates were able to come out of high school and walk right into a well-paying job. Within months of being hired, I would see many of them driving around in nice cars, living in nice apartments or well on their way to purchasing their first home.

My family was no different when it came to benefitting from the economic boom that was occurring in the city. We weren't rich, but I never missed a meal. We always had the essentials and a little something extra to be able to do things like take family vacations. This included frequently visiting my dad's family in Rome, Georgia or my mom's family in Roxboro, North Carolina. We also would do things like go to the movies. I was fortunate enough to take piano lessons for several years, and when I was around 10 years of age, I became a member of the Pioneer Girls which had a close resemblance to the Girl

Scouts. I can go on and on highlighting many of the amazing things about my birthplace. But it would suffice to say that Akron, Ohio was not only home, it was a great place to grow up.

Born on July 16, 1958 at Akron General Medical Center, I grew up feeling loved by both of my parents, but it was my mother who was actively involved in my child-rearing. This was because my father frequently was away from home for extended periods of time. And, when home, the majority of the time he worked as an entrepreneur using his skills and talents as a carpenter remodeling and installing siding on homes. As a result, he often did not have steady income.

My mother, therefore, was the major financial contributor to the household. She worked as a Telephone Operator for Ohio Bell. This was on top of her having to assume dual parental roles for my sister and me.

I do remember my father, during one period of time, having a 9 to 5 job. In fact, his first job was with the Ford Motor Company working at one of their plants. However, being an entrepreneur was my father's first love. So, on many occasions, he would call in sick from his regular job to complete his carpentry projects. This obviously added strain to my parent's relationship.

I truly felt my parents loved one another, but most of the time, I didn't see any expressions of affection between them. When I was very young, this didn't matter because I yearned the presence of my father and the positive energy and fun-loving attitude he always exuded. He had a calming presence and a certain style and sophistication about him, even in the way he dressed. He was such a good dresser that people who knew him would frequently say he was "dressed to the nines."

As I started getting older, into my preteen and teenage years, I slowly started to realize the emotional and physical toll their relationship was having on my mother. For years, I thought my father's extended absences were solely due to his work demands but later discovered that he frequently was gone for long stints due to infidelity.

I don't know what the tipping point was in their relationship, but they reached a place where they finally called it quits and my dad officially moved out. I believe it was due to a combination of my mother's growing independence and my father's desire to date other women. Knowing that she could not depend on my father, this bred a strong sense of independence in my mother. There was a certain toughness and resilience about her where she somehow always found a way to get things done.

The absence of my father left a tremendous void within me. I frequently would daydream about him walking through the front door. One particular day, when I was maybe nine or ten, my mom took us to the store. As we pulled into the parking lot of a shopping center on Arlington Road, who do I see? It's my father.

I yelled out "Mommy! Mommy! That's Daddy!"

I, then, ran up to his car, and he rolled down the window.

The first thing that caught my attention was how immaculately dressed he was. Then, before I could finish inspecting his full attire, I suddenly spotted someone else in the car. It was a woman.

Seeing her in the car totally caught me off guard. My entire body froze. I was speechless to the point that my jaw dropped, and my mouth remained wide open for several seconds. My father tried to play it off like the woman in the car was a colleague or that they were going to work or something. But, in my gut, I knew it was a lie.

A feeling of jealousy came over me seeing my father with another woman. This feeling of jealousy then quickly turned to resentment when I saw that the woman was wearing a gorgeous fur coat. I immediately wondered, "Did my father buy her that coat?"

Without question, the separation of my parents and witnessing events such as this had a profound effect on me. I wouldn't say it planted seeds of mistrust in men. It did, however, have an effect on my psychology about relationships or more so how I would define myself as a woman. Because of the kind of spirit I was born with, inevitably, I developed a loving heart and the capacity to deeply love a man. At the same time, I developed a mindset that I never wanted to be so dependent and reliant on a man, that I would not be able to take care of myself.

In other words, my childhood laid the foundation for my seeking a path in which I would not only be a wife and a mother, but I would also have a career. Psychologically, I just couldn't trust taking on the role of exclusively being a housewife.

Don't get me wrong. Nothing, absolutely nothing is wrong with this role. It just wasn't for me.

Becoming a Victim (My Most Painful Childhood Memory)

For most of the time that my parents were together, we lived in our own house or apartment. However, there was a period of time when my mom, dad, sister and I lived with my aunt and uncle.

Unfortunately, as loving as my uncle portrayed himself to be, he had a very dark side. He was a dirty old man, a child molester. He molested me on several occasions between the ages of five and seven. He would take me down into the basement so that he could look at me and touch me in inappropriate ways.

Amazingly, these horrible experiences never had a deeply traumatic impact on me. I had forgotten about them until the constant news reporting on this topic in the 90s caused some of these buried memories to resurface. By this time, I was already in my mid-30s, married and a mother of two.

There actually was a specific day in which I suddenly recalled many of the details from these past events. My mother, sister and I were sitting in the living room watching an episode of the Oprah Winfrey Show that focused on survivors of sexual abuse. It was a very engaging show given the subject matter. Oprah even shared on-camera her own personal experience of being sexually molested as a child.

At some point in the show, I had a gut reaction and blurted out, "That happened to me!!!" For some reason, hearing these stories and seeing these survivors stirred up all kinds of reactions and conversation among my mother, sister and me. We started sharing our own personal experiences with sexual abuse. This is how deeply embedded these memories were in my subconscious mind. I somehow had found a way to tuck them away and not allow them to affect my everyday life and emotional and mental state in any apparent way.

Fifty years later, I no longer view emotional wounding and vulnerability as a weakness. I no longer believe you should try to avoid, hide or run away from any painful memories from the past. Instead, I think you should tell someone and confront it head on. While I know feelings of shame, embarrassment, or even fear of the perpetrator retaliating, make it even more challenging to find someone you can trust talking to about these types of experiences, this is required as part of the healing process.

Outside of experiencing the separation of my parents and being sexually molested, my childhood overall was very positive. As previously expressed, I feel very blessed to have grown up in Akron, Ohio and to have been raised by my mother. There were many fun times and a strong sense of community and extended family—strong connections I maintain to this day.

I don't remember how long we lived with my aunt and uncle. I just remember abruptly moving out one day. My mother said it had to do with my aunt and her arguing about how my mother disciplined her kids. More specifically, on one occasion when my mother was about to reprimand me, my aunt—wanting to protect me from my mother—suddenly grabbed my mother's arm. For my mom, my great aunt responding in that way was a clear sign that it was time for us to find another place to live.

While living with my great aunt, the first elementary school I attended was Crouse Elementary. I loved that school. Then, when we moved into our own house again, we started attending Leggett Elementary. My sister and I rarely walked to school. Our mother would drive us to school and then pick us up at the end of the day.

Our house was located on Sherman street. The neighborhood we lived in was very vibrant, highly diverse and had a strong sense of community. Not at all typical of many communities in the 60s, both blacks and whites lived in our neighborhood and on the same street. We had white neighbors who lived right next to us and across the street from us. And, when it came to black and white kids playing together, this was not an issue at all. It was not frowned upon by any of our parents. They encouraged it. We frequently played at one friends' house who had a pet monkey.

Being Bullied

I was a pretty good student beginning as early as elementary. I always got "A's" and "B's." At the same time, I loved getting attention. So, I went out of my way to help and please the teacher. This, however, rubbed some students the wrong way. For this reason, my classmates referred to me as the teacher's pet.

Well, one particular time in 5th or 6th grade, there was a rumor going around that this girl, who was a very big girl for her age, was going to beat me up. Because I was not a fighter, I was scared to death walking home every day for at least a week straight. It was my sister who never had to worry about someone trying to bully her. Even though she was three years younger than me, because of her demeanor, no one ever tried to mess with her. My personality was one in which I tried to be everyone's friend and wanted everyone to like me. My sister, on the other hand, didn't care whether you liked her or not.

Finally, one day, when the girl confronted me in gym class, I didn't allow my fear to paralyze me. I really don't know what came over me, but I stood up to her. I guess I had just had enough. I said, "You know what? Just do it! Let's get it over with. I'm tired of you talking about me!!!" The only thought racing through my mind in that moment was "I'm not gonna let this girl beat me up."

The girl was taken aback. She obviously was not expecting that kind of reaction from me since I didn't have a reputation of being a fighter. To my surprise, she looked me dead in the eye and said, "I'm not gonna beat you up...." So, just like that, it was over. She never bothered me again.

I have no idea how much it had to do with my sister standing right there beside me when I was finally ready to fight. Because, there's no way my sister would have allowed that big girl to bully me or beat me up. However, it really didn't matter to me whether or not it was my sister's reputation that helped protect me in that situation. I was so proud of myself for finally having the courage to stand up for myself, to stand up to that bully. This was a life-changing moment for me to get in touch with a part of myself that I never knew existed—the fighter side of me that I had never tapped into before.

After that, I don't remember getting into any other fights or having any major conflicts with peers the entire time I matriculated through junior high and high school. This is because most of the kids I hung around, including my sister, were preoccupied with having fun, playing sports or other extracurricular activities, whether we were at school or at home.

I also, for the most part, steered clear of any kind of disciplinary issues. There, however, were a few times I was caught red handed doing something I knew I had no business doing. On occasion, I just couldn't resist the urge to be mischievous and to test boundaries.

One of these occasions was getting caught smoking cigarettes. My sister and I were left at home for the evening while our parents went out. We must have been in elementary school.

Our parents were never big smokers other than probably when they were out late with friends for special events. In fact, I don't think I ever saw my parents smoke my entire life. Well, anyway, that evening, we somehow stumbled across a pack of cigarettes. And, before we knew it, something possessed us to not only open the pack of cigarettes but to light a cigarette and start smoking it.

When we lit the cigarette, we really thought we were grown. You should have seen us. We were puffing and trying to blow smoke back out through our mouth. We were having a good ol' time until we heard the front door swing open. I turned to my sister nervously crying out to her "Put that cigarette out!!! Hurry up. They're coming!"

We were totally taken off guard and didn't have enough time to kill the smell from the cigarette smoke. We frantically sprayed air freshener but all it seemed to do was make the odor even stronger. That's when our mother walked into our room and yelled at us, "What are you doing!?!?" We quickly replied, "Nothing." She then responded, "Yes you are because I smell something."

Just like that, our moment of pure bliss turned into a living hell. My mother didn't play when it came to breaking rules or trying to think you're grown by lying to her or disrespecting her. So, when we said "Nothing" that just made her even more angry.

I assume you know what happened next. Well, the answer is, we got our butts beat. Incidences such as these, in which my mother resorted to physical discipline, led to nicknaming her "Zorro." It just wasn't that she knew how to handle a belt or a switch. She made it a demoralizing experience by telling you to go and find the switch that she would whoop you with.

One time I went to a tree in the backyard and got a switch. But my mom was like, "That ain't no switch!" She, then, went back outside and got a bigger switch and started removing the leaves so it would be skinny.

That was one of the worse whooping's ever. She tore my legs up. Given the color of my skin, you could see the red welts all of over my legs for hours.

Obviously, today, that would be called child abuse. But, in her defense, if she used a belt, it was always below the waist. She never hit us in the head, the face, the back or the chest. This is one thing I appreciate about my mother.

Additionally, now being a parent myself, I see the issue of disciplining your children from a totally different perspective than when I was a kid. As a parent, I also strongly believe that children should have some level of fear of their parents so that they will think twice before making bad or poor decisions; fear is intertwined with respect.

Once again, outside of a few incidences of mischief, I generally was well-behaved. As a very happy-go-lucky person, I was always in search of fun and having a good time with my family and friends. This is why I always looked forward to going to our other Great Uncle Joe and Great Aunt Lillian's house. This aunt was my maternal grandmother's sister. Whenever we went there, we were guaranteed to have fun. We spent so much time there that it became like a second home to us. We would spend the night or stay over for days at a time.

One of the most hilarious things my sister and I would do during visits was to put on concerts. We literally would rehearse songs and sing and dance like we were professional artists. There would be different themes ranging from Gospel to Elvis impersonations.

Other fun things we did at their house were playing tennis at Edgewood Courts directly across the street from their house or going to the Akron Zoo which also was nearby. They had a dog named Smokey who looked like a Rottweiler but had a tail. He would keep us company by laying at the foot of our bed anytime we spent the night.

Then, of course, every Sunday after church, we ate dinner at their house. Some of my favorites were fried chicken, roast beef, mac and cheese, black eyed peas, yams (sweet potatoes), and greens. Her cornbread was to die for. I think it's because she used buttermilk.

This aunt really pushed us to consistently attend church. We were with her so much that naturally we had to tag along. Her home church was Coburn Street Church of God at 807 Coburn Street.

I was nine years old in elementary school at the time. We quickly became active members which meant joining the choir, being in the youth ministry and frequently attending church more than once a week. One of the most significant things to happen as a result of being a member of the Coburn Street Church of God is that this is where I met my High School Sweetheart.

Our introduction to one another was not "love at first sight." We actually had been members of the same church for five years before he ever expressed any interest. Then, one day, when I was 14 years old and he was 15, he just walked up to me out of nowhere, while I was coming out of church, and asked for my phone number. Once I realized who it was, I was like, "Really, my number??? Oh, okay. Sure..."

Never before had I considered dating him. I was so crazy and love struck over another member of the church who was a few years older than me. And, when I say young man, I mean young man. Technically, because he was about five years older than me, I never should have been trying to talk to him. However, he was so fine I didn't care. I had such a crush on him that I was willing to suffer the consequences.

I used to just stare at him and his gorgeous hair while sitting in church. I assumed he had no interest in me whatsoever until one day he gave me a beautiful Blue Stone broach for Christmas. All this did was make matters worse and even more confusing for me because nothing ever came of it. He never asked me for my number. So, we never went on a date or even talked on the phone.

To say the least, my new pursuer had stiff competition to overcome. Nonetheless, he made such an impression on me after our first phone conversation that I became equally interested in him from then on. Adding fuel to the fire, I was very bold for my age. I didn't sit around waiting for his call. Despite knowing that it was taboo for girls to call boys, especially teenage girls at that, I would call him first. This would be right after school or sometimes in the evening. Then, as soon as he would answer the phone, I would tell him to call me right back so that it would appear as though he was calling me.

We would talk on the phone for hours at a time. As a result, we grew closer and closer. Within a few short months, our relationship progressed to the point where we were being chaperoned by my mother to different church and community events, like church youth functions. Because I wasn't allowed to officially date until I was 16, this was the only way we were allowed to spend quality time together outside of church.

My mom drove us from place to place, with my sister tagging along. He and I would sit in the backseat of the car. This way it was not considered "official" dating. He was more like a family friend.

He and I developed deep feelings for one another to the point of saying that we were in love. We had a phrase that was a play on words: *'I evol you'* – That's LOVE spelled backwards.

One of the sweetest and most romantic things he ever did for me was throw me a surprise party for my Sweet 16th Birthday. Turning 16 was the big moment I had eagerly been waiting for. He would finally be able to take me out to dinner somewhere nice as a couple without adults chaperoning us. These plans were abruptly put on hold when he suffered a serious injury at work where he nearly cut off his finger working on a machine. He was employed by a Lumber Company that built windows. He was good at working with wood. The injury was so severe that he had to go to the hospital. Because of his injury, I assumed there was no way he would be in good enough health to still go out on a date.

The day of my birthday, already expecting to be locked in the house instead of out having fun, I was surprised to receive a call from his twin brother. When I answered, he said, *"I know my brother was supposed to take you out, but I'm gonna have to take you out instead."* Not having anything else to do, and not wanting to be stuck in the house on my birthday, I gladly accepted the invitation.

I had no idea where we were going. I just found it very strange that his twin brother kept stopping at payphones every 30 minutes or so to make a phone call. It wasn't until later that I put two and two together and realized that he kept stopping to call the house where my surprise party was being held. He wanted to make sure we didn't arrive there too soon. His twin brother was just driving me around as a distraction to buy some time until all the guests arrived at my friend's house where the surprise party was being held.

At some point, his twin finally said, 'Let's go see a friend'. I said "Sure." Because she was a good friend of ours, I still had no clue of what was going on.

When we arrived and walked through the front door of my friend's house, she immediately directed us to head downstairs to the basement. Upon reaching the bottom of the stairs, I looked up and lo' and behold "Who do I see?" It was my boo surrounded by at least thirty close friends and family members. I was in total shock that after suffering a major injury, he found the energy and the time to organize and plan the entire surprise party. I was deeply touched and moved by this gesture. I thought it was so sweet of him.

The next year of my life and our relationship seemed to fly by. Before I knew it, I was heading off to college.

While he and I remained closer than ever, we were starting to be confronted with new challenges in our relationship. As a result, we experienced our first breakup. Actually, I broke up with him after attending a revival at church. For several days, the pastor had been preaching on the significance of being "equally yoked" in intimate relationships, and even more in marriage. I was so transfixed by the sermons that to this day I can still remember the Bible verses he cited: II Corinthians 6:14 ESV – *"Do not be unequally yoked with unbelievers. For what partnership has righteousness with lawlessness? Or what fellowship has light with darkness?"*

The pastor's message struck me so hard that I began to question whether he and I were equally yoked. I literally said to him, "We have to break up because we're not equally yoked." He looked at me like I was crazy.

I didn't have any concern for how this would impact him emotionally. I was most concerned with doing what I felt was the "Will of God". Therefore, I had no sense of tact or etiquette. I didn't care about breaking it to him lightly. I just wanted to relieve myself of any feelings of guilt or possibly living in sin.

It wasn't until after I did it that I clearly knew I went about it the wrong way. I at least could have or should have talked to him face-to-face instead of just breaking up with him over the phone. The damage, however, was done. I had crushed him. I had broken his heart.

You'll probably laugh when you hear this. But, it probably wasn't more than a couple of weeks before we were right back together. Our connection was so strong that it was just too difficult for us to be apart. Our emotions had gone to such a deep level that we weren't ready to let go of the relationship and to officially call it quits.

Another very interesting twist was that, in the process of reconciling, he shared with me that before I broke up with him, he was about to propose to me. He told me that he had already picked out a ring. Even though I was just weeks away from heading off to college, he said he didn't care. He already knew that he wanted us to be husband and wife.

Lessons on Childhood Experiences

1. Don't let people bully you. Or, if you're being bullied, tell someone. This is an important lesson not just for us adults but for teaching our children.

2. Don't be afraid to tell someone who is trying to harm you "NO" even if the perpetrator threatens you and/or your family.

3. If child molestation is still haunting you as an adult, have the courage to seek help to begin and/or continue the process of healing.

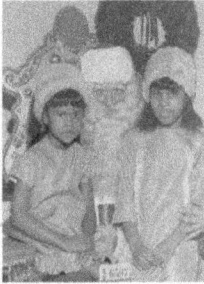
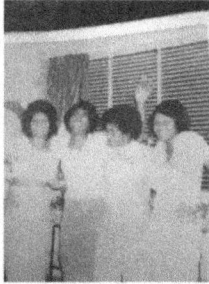
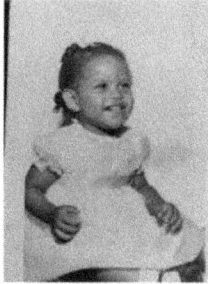

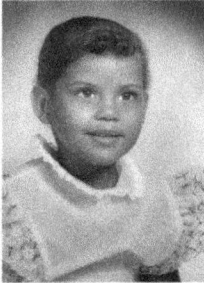
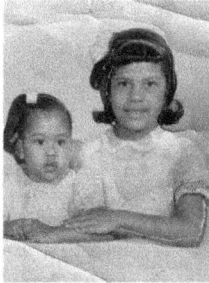
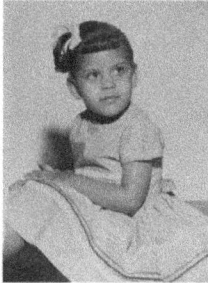

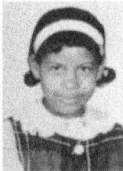
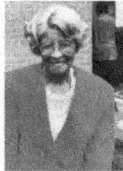
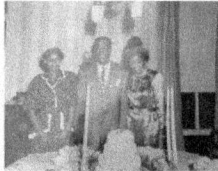
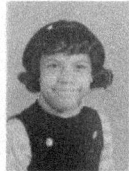

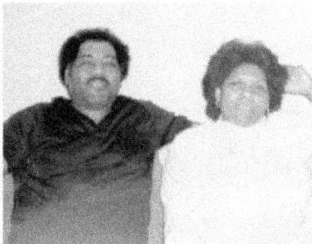
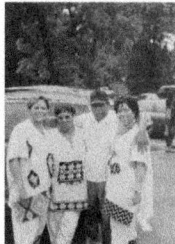
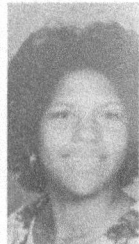

CHAPTER 2
FINDING MY CAREER PATH

Going Off to College

The college I chose to attend was Mount Union College just 45 minutes southeast of Akron, Ohio. I was far enough away to feel as though I had taken a major leap into adulthood and at the same time was still close enough to be able to consistently see my family and friends. Because of the close proximity, I probably came home every other weekend.

Mount Union was a predominantly white private school. While I had grown up in a very diverse community, I still experienced a certain degree of culture shock. As a private school, many of the students came from very affluent families. Fortunately, despite the adjustments I had to make socially and mentally, my grades did not suffer. I made a relatively smooth transition from high school to college.

The most perplexing thing that happened to me one year was this upper classman liked me and I didn't know it. We had freshman orientation and they assigned each freshman to an upperclassman. I was assigned to Tulip and she was a few years older than me. Anyway, it was their responsibility to show us around campus and help us get adjusted to college life. She was a part of the girls' softball team and I played tennis and volleyball. However, she convinced me to also join the softball team.

She would always come to our room, and as softball season progressed, I remember some of the girls would sit rather close to each other. This and a number of other things I began to notice led me to believe many of them liked each other. Tulip would spend more and more time in our room, but she never made a pass at me. I just thought it was strange her conversation would never be about boys. Unlike many of my other friends on campus, our conversations always centered around boys.

Anyway, one of the baseball players came up to me and said, "You do know that Tulip likes you, that's why she's always hanging around you?" I was like, "WHAT?" "NO!" I was totally shocked and devasted at the same time by the thought that a girl could be physically and sexually attracted to me.

Well, a month or so later, it was time for one of the holidays or breaks and Tulip asked if she could come home with me because she lived far away. I said, "Yes." But, this way before I found out she liked me. Anyway, it was close to the day I was going to leave for break, and I told my roommate that I needed to talk to Tulip so that I could tell her she could not come home with me. I told my roommate to leave, but to check on me, just in case the conversation didn't go well.

Tulip came to my room and I told her she couldn't come home with me. I probably made up a story. Immediately after giving her the news, I could see she was hurt. After that, she never hung out in our room again and we would just acknowledge each other with a nod when we saw each other on campus. I eventually quit the softball team and just focused on Tennis and Volleyball.

Believe it or not, the greatest challenge I had to contend with was during my sophomore year of college. It was the rapidly changing dynamics in my relationship with my first love. With each day that passed, the dynamics of our relationship became more and more bittersweet. We found ourselves in a perpetual cycle of breaking up, making up, and getting back together again.

One time, he broke up with me saying, "I think we should see other people." Shortly thereafter, I discovered that he broke up with me to go with another girl. To make matters worse, I later also found out that he went to the same high school as his new girlfriend. She was a few years younger than him. To say the least, I was totally devastated.

This kind of stuff continued to happen repeatedly over and over again. One day I remember coming back to my dorm room and being greeted by my roommate and one of her friends. I kept a picture of him hanging up on the wall close to my bed. The friend of my roommate out of nowhere says, "Isn't that such and such's boyfriend?"

It took me a minute to replay in my mind what I had just heard. Then, once what she had said fully computed in my mind, I turned to her and said, "Can you repeat what you just said?"

She turned to me and restated, "Isn't that such and such's boyfriend?" I angrily replied, "No way! That's my boyfriend!!!"

Even though the girl knew she was telling the truth about him having two girlfriends at once, she didn't push the issue because she could see how angry and hurt I was.

Another layer of pain was inflicted just a few days later when I found out his new girl was a friend of one of his cousins.

Cheater, cheater, cheater. Everyone kept telling me to let him go and move on. However, this was much easier said than done. We had what I guess you would call a "Codependent Relationship" even though this was a term that was rarely used, if at all, back then. Despite the pleading from my friends, and even my mother telling me to let him go, we kept holding on to each other. We continued the cycle of breaking up and making up.

It got so bad and I was so miserable that I could not stop crying for days at a time. It was like a spell was cast over me. I tried everything imaginable to let go and move on from the relationship, but nothing worked. This included fasting and praying out loud to God, "Lord if it is not meant for us to be together, please take my desire for him away from my heart! Please Lord give me the strength to move on!" Then, within just 24 hours of starting my fasting and praying, he called and apologized saying he was sorry, that he loved me, and wanted to be with ONLY ME! Just like that, we were right back together again.

In the midst of being on this emotional rollercoaster, a life-changing opportunity presented itself. The Fortune 500 company Rubbermaid came to Mount Union College to interview students. They were looking to fill a number of internship positions. For any student who landed one of these internships, it basically meant they were guaranteeing themselves a great job immediately following graduation. And, at that time, I was in my junior year.

I passed the first interview which was held on our campus. I, then, was invited to a second interview at the corporate offices of Rubbermaid which was in Wooster, Ohio. This was about a forty-five minute to an hour drive from the Mount Union campus in Alliance, Ohio. I nailed the interview and, just a few days later, I was given an official offer letter.

Initially, the internship was supposed to be a rotating schedule of going to school for 3 months, working for 3 months, going to school for 3 months, working for 3 months and so on. So, instead of graduating in 4 years, I would graduate in 5 years. Things, however, got even better. After the first 3 months of my internship, Rubbermaid was so pleased with my work that they offered me a job making $18,000 a year. In 1980, this was an unbelievable salary for a college student!

My mother, however, had mixed feelings about my taking on a full-time job while still in school. She feared that I would fall in love with the money and not graduate. So, she made me promise that I would stay in school and complete my degree. Fortunately, Mount Union College (now called the University of Mount Union) allowed me to remain a full-time student while working full-time. It just meant that I would have to become a non-traditional student at Mount Union. This required me to move off-campus and start meeting with my professors at their homes to turn in my assignments. When it was time for me to take classes, my mom would ride with me to my professor's house. My new place of residence was in the home of an elderly lady who had a room for rent in Wooster, Ohio. It was about a five-minute drive to Rubbermaid.

My first official work assignment was in Rubbermaid's Accounting department. But somehow, at the last minute, they ended up moving me to the Research department. Here, I was able to see firsthand how the company made many of its new products. In this department, I also learned how surveys and research analysis were conducted.

Another added responsibility during my internship was serving as a Research Coordinator. This required me to hire college students from nearby Wooster College as well as adults from the local community. Frequently, it would be housewives looking for part-time work.

As Research Coordinator, I was responsible for getting feedback by asking the general public to complete surveys on current products or by displaying models of prototypes and products getting ready for future production. We would go to various locations throughout the greater Akron area and setup tables at malls. We would then administer surveys with consumers to find out which products they would like to see come to market. We would conduct these surveys a few times a month.

Every day I went to work it felt like I was learning something new. I never knew these types of specialty departments existed within companies. I loved it!

On one occasion, I remember doing research on what would be the best size and shape for the plastic container of a new product that was being launched. Some of the questions we asked were: Should it be round? Rectangle? Clear? Opaque? I also would go to various retail outlets like K-Mart, purchase all of our competitors' plasticware and bring them back to the Rubbermaid offices to compare prices, sizes and durability.

I even had the opportunity to travel out of state to a "Color Conference in Orlando, Florida." This is where you could learn about the psychological and subconscious implications of using certain colors when making products and when marketing them. You also saw first-hand, colors of the future. When I returned from the conference, I was so full of ideas that Rubbermaid allowed me to contribute and make recommendations on the colors for a new kitchen line.

Lessons on Finding Your Career Path

1. College may not be for everyone. So, don't beat yourself up if you don't feel motivated to take that path. What is important is to find a path where you can make the kind of living you want to make and enjoy going to work every day.

2. Once you figure out what you want to do, or what you're passion about, take the first step in learning about and educating yourself on that particular career path or profession (make sure you get the credentials needed to set yourself up for success).

3. Start by making a list of your interests, and better yet things that you are passionate about and would do for free because you enjoy it that much.

4. Set some goals for your career path: short-term and long-term.

CHAPTER 3
MARRIAGE

He Proposes

Holding down a full-time job and going to school full-time was draining but exhilarating. In so many facets of my work I was gaining real-world experience that I knew was invaluable. On top of that, I still was going back and forth to Akron to see my man. He had a one-bedroom apartment on Arlington Road.

I remember coming home one evening or weekend to attend a revival at church. So, I stopped by his apartment because we were going to ride together to church. When I went into his apartment, he had his coat on but was just sitting there on the couch. I said "Honey. What are you doing? Aren't you ready to go?"

He said, "Do you love me?"

I said, "Yeah. Of course... Now, come on. We are going to be late for church."

He didn't budge. He, instead, motioned for me to come sit next to him on the couch.

Then, just like that he blurted out, "Will you marry me?"

The moment I heard those words and saw the ring in his hand I screamed loud enough for everyone in his apartment building to hear me. I don't remember if it was before or after church, but we went from house to house announcing the news that we were getting married.

Given our history of constantly breaking up and my being an emotional wreck time and time again, overloading family and friends with our emotional relationship drama, my mother was not excited for us. She wasn't trying to rain on our parade. She just had witnessed the whole sequence of events from when we were teenagers to now as young adults still trying to reach a point or place in our relationship where it was totally smooth sailing. She, therefore, felt – and for good reason – that we were making a big mistake to be talking about marriage at such a young age.

My mother liked him as a person because he had become a part of the family. But, she did not have confidence in him as a mate for me especially since most of the times that we broke up it was over a girl. And, I would cry a lot. My mom, just like any parent or loved one, hated seeing me cry.

Nevertheless, we proceeded with the wedding arrangements and were married a year later on July 28, 1979. We had 12 bridesmaids and groomsmen and two ministers perform the ceremony which was held at our home church where we met as children.

We moved into his one-bedroom apartment, and I continued to work at Rubbermaid. I was just 21. Two years later I graduated from college. Out of respect for my mother, I kept my family name of Delphyne Turner Lomax on my diploma. Less than a year after graduating, we purchased our first home. It was an old three-story house on Manchester Road. I think we paid $21,000 for it and the monthly mortgage payment was only $270. After we moved in, I remember the man across the street saying we probably could have gotten it for $18,000.

I look back now and think, "Wow! We paid only $18,000 for our first house. Those where the days, because twenty years later, we bought the house I now live in for around $120,000. Although, I must admit that back then we were talking about a 70-year-old house with 3 bedrooms and 1 bathroom, not a new house with 5 bedrooms and 3 bathrooms.

Marriage

Marriage is one of the most sacred things in life. Well, at least, that's my opinion. My belief is that God made man and woman to be a team, to be joined together and to create, or to procreate that is. Therefore, marriage and family go hand-in-hand.

It is true that my strong religious background has heavily influenced my beliefs and perspectives on marriage and family. The fact that I got married at a young age has also significantly contributed to the shaping of my beliefs. What if I, for example, had waited to get married in my mid to late 30s as opposed to my early 20s? Who knows what beliefs and thoughts about marriage and family I would have held on to so many years later in life? To say the least, I entered into marriage with a mindset firmly fixated on fulfilling the marital vow of "Til' death do us part" and "Happily ever after."

For 30+ years of my life, my only sexual partner was my husband. I only share such intimate details to emphasize the point I'm trying to make. That is, for over three decades of my life, everything in my life revolved around my marriage. This was my greatest priority.

When I was at work, I was thinking about being at home with my husband. When I got home, I immediately thought about what my husband wanted for dinner. I literally attended to his every need, not only cooking but washing clothes, cleaning the house, and so on.

The beauty of it was that, because I was in love, none of this felt like work to me. I not only saw it as my Godly duty and responsibility as a wife to take care of my husband and the house. I wanted to do it because it felt good doing it.

I was not only madly in love with my husband. He was my childhood sweetheart. Even though we tried countless times to break up, it just never happened. Now that we were married, I was all in. I had big hopes and dreams of building an amazing life together, of starting and having a family.

Lessons on Marriage

1. Communication must be a high priority! You've gotta make sure you communicate the "good" and the "bad," your likes and your dislikes. Always keep in mind that No one is or should be expected to be a mind reader. And it doesn't matter if you've been married one year or fifty years, two-way communication is important.

2. For those who are married, and have extended their family with children, remember to nurture your relationship and not solely focus on your children.

3. Date Night is a great way you and your partner can spend significant and consistent quality time together. This is a helpful tool or rule to live by especially for couples who have very busy and hectic schedules.

4. We know arguments and disagreements can happen in relationships. Be extra cautious in deciding who is mature enough to give you sound, balanced and unbiased advice and guidance.

5. Finances: We all need money to live. If you aren't on the same page with your partner, it is a major contender for tearing a great relationship apart. So, make the first priority to be responsible and accountable yourself for the financial decisions you make as an individual and as a team.

6. Don't be complacent with your relationship. After 10 years of being in a relationship, for example, many couples forget what initially brought them together. What initially made them fall in love with each other? Never lose that.

CHAPTER 4
MOTHERHOOD

Having Children

We had been married 3 years when we had our first son, Dale II. In fact, I had just turned 24. I clearly remember, in the month of July, getting the news that I was pregnant. This is because we were preparing to celebrate our 3rd wedding anniversary.

Dale II was born on March 20, 1982 at 7:48pm at Akron General Hospital. There was nothing out of the ordinary on that Saturday. As we customarily did, we spent the entire day making our rounds visiting with family and friends. Late in the day, while at my mother-in-law's house on the North side of town (Turner Street), I suddenly started having pains. The pains were so intense that even when everyone ordered pizza, I decided not to eat.

Over the next hour, the increased throbbing in my abdomen continued every 30 minutes, and then every 15 to 20 minutes. We called my doctor's office and they instructed us to go straight to the hospital. We were somewhat unprepared as the baby was not expected to arrive for a few more weeks. We didn't even have a bag packed. Our baby's due date was not until March 24th.

Arriving at the hospital, we checked in and were quickly seen by a doctor. Some of the first words I can recall hearing the medical team communicate back and forth were, "She's almost a 10.... fully dilated." And, they were periodically urging me to "Hold it! Don't Push! Hold it!"

The other events that occurred from then on in the delivery room may not occur as frequently today as they did back in the 80s. That is, men (the father of the child) could be in the delivery room the entire time. My husband did just that. He was by my side every single moment holding my hand and trying his best to comfort me.

Together, we had been preparing for the birth of our first child by taking child birthing classes. Yet, when the reality and truth of the moment hit us — that we were having a baby — all of our training and preparation went right out the window. When those labor pains started getting up to a Level 10 and we started trying to utilize all the techniques and strategies we had learned in Lamaze classes, nothing seemed to work. I'm definitely not saying my husband wasn't supportive because he was fully supportive. It's just that everything was happening so fast that we were caught up in a whirlwind.

Everyone was constantly checking on me and my husband. He was holding my hand, and I was squeezing his hands very tightly. Then, when one of my cousins showed up, she kept rubbing my arm to try and keep me calm. She thought she was comforting me. All the while, I was thinking to myself "Please stop rubbing my arm!" Despite it being such an intense situation, I somehow kept my cool to not blurt out to her what I was thinking.

One technique or relaxation strategy from the child birthing classes that actually did work in the moment was trying to find a focal point, something you can fixate on. Lying there in the midst of all this chaos, I somehow remembered this technique and tried it. A coat hanger or coat hook on the back of the door on the other side of the room caught my attention and I locked in on it.

The timing of using this technique was perfect because the pain had become excruciating. By now, I was not only physically exhausted. I was mentally and emotionally exhausted. People were constantly bombarding me with questions and trying to tell me what to do. I just wanted it to be over.

Rolling me down the hall and back into the Delivery Room one staff member was saying "Breathe!" Another person was saying "Push!" Then, another one was saying "Stay relaxed!"

This was so frustrating because my instinct was to push the baby out as quickly as possible with the hope of finally being able to alleviate the pain. The doctors, however, were saying just the opposite. They kept telling me to wait, "Don't Push!". In the meanwhile, I just tried to keep a steady rhythm of inhaling and exhaling (hee hee hee hee whoooooo .... hee hee hee hee whooooo....). Not having been sedated, I reached a breaking point where I just couldn't hold it any longer and instinctively pushed despite the medical staff urging me not to because, the doctor was about to give me an episiotomy, that is, a surgical cut made at the opening of the vagina during childbirth. This brought on even more pain as I tore open my lower section to the point I later had to be stitched back together.

Everything that occurred after that is a blur. I only remember being greeted with an unforgettable moment of joy. This is the moment when I saw my firstborn come into this world. Our physician, yelled out, with a big smile on his face, "It's a Boy!!!"

My husband, all in the same instance, released my hand, which he had been holding off and on for several hours. Without saying a word, he exited the delivery room. Family and friends later reported to me that he paced up and down the hall yelling "I got myself a boy!!! I got myself a boy!!!"

We both were so excited. There had been a big buildup to this moment especially since we had no idea if it would be a boy or a girl. Back in the day, having an ultrasound to determine the gender of the baby was not standard procedure.

Moments later, when my husband tried to get back into the room to share this moment with me, they denied him access. This was due to the increased possibility of infection because he was no longer sterile.

Our baby boy was 8 pounds, 8 ounces. We named him Dale Kerry Lomax II. It was such a special moment that I held on to a few mementos. One of them is the little wrist band they give you once you are born and admitted into the baby ward in the hospital.

Returning home with an infant changed the energy in our home and the dynamics of our husband-wife relationship. Our newborn was clearly the focal point. He was not only adored and cared for by us. There were countless family members and friends who pitched in to help. We truly had a village assisting us.

Fortunately, I didn't have to rush back to work. I stayed home for an entire 6 weeks, and it was wonderful. Another major blessing, once I returned to work, was not having to pay for daycare because my mom offered to watch him. This lasted for at least the next couple of years.

While I had the luxury of being on maternity leave for 6 weeks, and was surrounded by plenty of support, there still were a few rough moments learning how to be a mom. On one occasion, I locked my child in the car. It occurred while I was on my way to a friend's baby shower. I had preplanned all the details of packing a diaper bag, a purse and other essentials. Then, just like that, while trying to gather all my stuff out of the front seat and lock the door at the same, I turned and without realizing it, the door slammed shut. I forgot that my keys were still in the car. "Thank God," with new cars, you can't leave your key in the ignition and lock the door. It won't lock or you will hear a constant beep.

Once I realized I locked my keys in the car, a sense of panic instantly came over me. I screamed out "Oh my God, I just locked my baby in the car!!!"

Then, out of nowhere, this man appeared. My protective instinct tried to take hold of me by attempting to quickly assess if I could trust him to help me in this dire situation. He could be a criminal for all I knew. Before I could be too critical or judgmental of his character, my mind also quickly processed that the other alternative to trusting this stranger was continuing to watch my child being locked inside the car while I stood there helplessly.

So, in some non-verbal way, I think I just nodded to the gentleman "You have my permission. Go ahead and do what you have to do." And, just like that, he jimmied the door and the door was opened within seconds.

There definitely were other stressful moments in learning to be a parent, but I never did anything like that again. I quickly learned to be alert and more attentive at all times. One significant thing that greatly helped was, for the most part, I was hardly ever alone. Help always seemed to be nearby. This was partly due to having such a strong knit family. It was also due to the fact that there were very few infants in our family.

I do need to take a pause here and say that on my husband's side of the family his twin brother had a baby that was very pre-mature. I will never forget going to the hospital pregnant with Lil Dale and my sister-in-law going into labor three months early and had him. Lil Donald stayed in the hospital for 3 months fighting for his life. My nephew is now an adult, married with children of his own. Ain't God good!

Okay, back to the story .... On my side of the family, my sister didn't have children at the time. Even though my in-laws had 8 children, Dale II along with Donald II were among the youngest grandchildren at the time. They were the babies, and everyone gravitated to them. Before we knew it, he was being spoiled to death.

Once, when I had to go out of town for a conference for work, we made it a family vacation and took Baby Dale (that's what some people still call him to this day). That's when things shifted for my mother as a caretaker. It was during our time away that my mother realized how much more rest she was getting without him being around. So, when we returned from our trip, my mother said it was time to find someone else to watch him.

I believe the next person to look after him was Irma Jones Day Care. We got lucky once again because we lived on Manchester Road, and Irma Jones Day Care was right around the corner. Those working at Irma Jones loved watching after Dale, but we always had to make sure he had enough milk, in just the right kind of cup, along with a piece of cheese. If you didn't have these exact items: the cheese and the milk in the right cup, Baby Dale, would have a fit. There would be an all-out non-stop crying tantrum.

Being a mother and raising a son was great. Even though juggling a 9 to 5 job, then coming home to tend to my infant while also being a wife to my husband, made for a very busy life, I was extremely happy. We were surrounded by loving family and friends which meant our child was being raised in an amazing environment of extended family and a strong sense of community.

We didn't have another child right away. It was another three years before we had our second son Daniel. Being somewhat comfortable financially we wanted more than one kid, it was somewhat planned. At the same time, my husband and I weren't totally on the same page about exactly how many kids we should have. To put it bluntly, he wanted to have a football team and I was fine with just three or four. However, when Daniel was born, the decision about how many kids we would have was settled once and for all. I wasn't having any more kids. It was just too painful, and I didn't want to go through it anymore. Besides, two seemed like enough; a family of four was alright with us.

The day before Daniel was born, I started having severe cramps. Having already given birth to my first child, I had been mentally prepared to endure a certain amount of pain. But this time, I was experiencing a different kind of physical discomfort. The cramps really started to intensify around 11pm. That's when I told my husband we needed to head to the hospital. He called my mother to come over and watch Baby Dale. Once she arrived, we immediately headed out the door.

When we arrived at the hospital, they said I was like a 2. For people who are unfamiliar with child birthing medical terminology, you need to be dilated at a 10 for them to feel that you're almost ready to give birth. I, however, refused to go home. Despite what my physical symptoms were indicating medically, I just knew in my gut that it was time. Every part of my being mentally, emotionally and spiritually was just ready to have that baby—especially since I was feeling a certain sense of resolve that this was the last time, I was going to have a baby. Simply stated in plain English "I was done!

The medical staff finally relented to my wishes and they induced labor. Shortly thereafter, they broke my water. Amazingly, my time in labor was nowhere near close to the typical 12, 16, or 18 hours. It literally seemed like I went into the hospital and came right back out with a baby boy.

During my short stay in the hospital, I still found enough time to make sure my tubes were tied. My husband had no problems signing the necessary paperwork. I don't know if it's like that today, but in the 80's if you were married, your husband had to consent to you having your tubes tied. So much for it being the woman's body – huh!

Daniel was born on a Saturday morning at 6:43AM (March 12, 1985). He was 7 pounds and 7 ounces. What made his birth extra special is that his father's birthday is March 13 and his older brother Dale II Birthday is March 20th. So, we have three birthday celebrations in the month of March.

Upon my release from the hospital, I enjoyed another extended maternity leave. Again, I stayed home from work for 6 weeks. Just like Baby Dale, I breastfed Daniel and used the pump. When I returned to work, I continued to do both for probably another month or so.

While we deeply loved our second child, there definitely wasn't the same level of enthusiasm as having our first child. I really felt bad for Daniel. He wasn't spoiled in the same way Dale II was. Again, once I went back to work, I only nursed Daniel for a few more weeks. After that, I said, 'That's it! I'm done buddy."

It's like some kind of psychological shift occurred within me as well as within my husband. I mean even simple things like taking pictures. We just didn't have the same energy level and motivation as we did with our first born. When you look at our photo albums there's tons of pictures of Baby Dale. We took enough pictures to capture every little moment: at 6 weeks; at 3 months; at 6 months; at 9 months; at 12 months. Even our son Daniel, once he got older, realized this huge discrepancy in the number of pictures we had of him compared to how many pictures we had of his older brother.

While celebrating the birth of our second child, we also were greeted with some bad news. My husband's job at the Murphy Lumber Company had been rock solid in terms of providing a steady and decent paycheck. For reasons unknown, the company suddenly started going through a period of layoffs and these cutbacks weren't expected to end anytime soon.

Constantly worrying about whether he would be laid off started to weigh on us. As a result, we began thinking about moving to another city that would provide greater job opportunities and greater overall job security. At the top of our list was Atlanta. Or, should I say the city of Lithonia.

While Murphy Lumber Company significantly reduced my husband's work hours for extended periods of time, he was never fully laid off. This, however, was enough to convince us that it definitely was time for a change. In the spring of 1985, while I was still pregnant with Daniel, my husband moved to Atlanta when a more stable job opportunity opened up. He landed a job helping my father in construction and lived with one of my cousins.

My husband would come back to Akron as often as he could. However, it got to the point where he missed us terribly and came back to Akron. I clearly remember him saying, "I am not going back to Atlanta unless we are all together." So, within a few months of Daniel being born, we made the decision to move to Atlanta. At the time, Daniel was 5 months old and Dale II was 3.

Our relocation to Atlanta (Lithonia, Georgia) was relatively smooth despite neither one of us having a job when we first arrived. The one good thing was that we already had daycare in place because my cousin, who was a stay-at-home mom, had eagerly agreed to watch both of our sons. Since she was already raising her only child Stacy, she just agreed to take on Dale and Daniel.

She later secured a part-time job. With this new schedule, she would watch the three kids for part of the day before heading off to work. My cousin would drop Stacy off at La Petit childcare and Dale and Daniel attended a KinderCare daycare center right near our apartment complex (Alexandria Apartments).

Once Dale started attending Elementary School, I became very active in the PTA. I also would chaperone on some of the school field trips. I even enrolled both of them in an organization called "The Winning Circle." The organizer would come to the school and talk about self-esteem and other character-building traits. He also had a drill team. Though mainly for boys, the organization later was opened to girls to participate in all the various activities.

Being a part of the Winning Circle required a significant commitment of time. There were a number of fundraising activities including an annual banquet in which different community leaders were recognized for their work in child advocacy. This is why the organization was called the "The Winning Circle."

The tireless work of the organizer and the overall Winning Circle program model was very powerful and highly impactful. It was a great organization for Dale and Daniel as well as other kids throughout the community.

One-character trait we repeatedly emphasized with them was to always be truthful, to never lie. Another trait was to always be respectful to adults, to teachers and authority figures. We told our sons that when an adult, or anyone for that matter, was speaking to them to always look them in the face. While we didn't raise our kids to say 'Yes, ma'am" or "No, ma'am', we quickly discovered that this was a big deal in the south. For many native southerners in the late 80s, if you didn't say "Ma'am" or "Sir," you were being disrespectful. There were very clear lines that were not to be crossed when it came to showing respect to authority figures.

One time an issue of respect came into play with one of the teachers at Daniels school when he was in kindergarten or first grade. He kept telling us a teacher was always picking on him. This particular teacher was a short Caucasian lady and had a totally different perspective of what was taking place. She alleged that Daniel had violated her space. However, when I got feedback from other staff at the school who pulled me to the side to let me know they had witnessed the incident, they reported to me that Daniel was not disruptive at all. After hearing this, I immediately called a meeting with Daniel's teacher.

Meeting in her classroom at the school, the three of us sat in a circle. Taking control of the meeting, I quickly started off by saying, "So, he did what?"

That's when the teacher started stuttering. The only words she could utter were, Nothing.... Nothing..." To say the least, she was totally speechless.

I, however, did not let her off the hook that easily. I continued by specifically asking her, "Did you say he violated your space? How is that possible when he is in kindergarten? He doesn't know anything about boundaries!"

I got her all tongue tied and scared and nervous to the point that she ended up apologizing directly to Daniel.

For me, this was a very proud moment—not because I came out on the winning side and got the teacher to apologize. Because, I affirmed to my son the importance of being respectful to others while at the same time teaching him that he should never be ashamed of or allow anyone to be disrespectful to him, not even adults. Secondly, I was letting him know, at a very early age, that I will always have his back whenever he chooses to do the right thing. These are two major life lessons that were reinforced with my children throughout their childhood and even now as adults.

As my boys progressed through elementary and onto middle school, I really became frustrated with the restructuring of the middle school and high school grade levels. For years, high school was 10th through 12th grade. Then, for some strange reason, school districts started changing middle school to 6th through 8th grade and high school became 9th through 12th grade.

I really hate this grade level system. In my opinion, 7th grade is a great time to transition to middle school, but 9th grade is just too early to be transitioning to high school.

As previously stated, I've always been actively involved in my children's lives and so was my husband. While I thought I was doing an amazing job, there's one piece of advice my mother gave me when my children were ages 10 and 7. This advice significantly shifted my focus and approach to parenting. My mother's statement was that our children needed to be more physically active not just being busy bodies participating in a bunch of clubs and extra academic classes. In heeding her advice, we enrolled our sons in a basketball program at the South DeKalb Family YMCA and then I started volunteering for the local branch and Headquarters of the Metropolitan Atlanta YMCA.

Our affiliation with the YMCA has continued for more than twenty-five years. The YMCA is where my sons first started playing sports and discovered their love of basketball. It provided a highly structured environment where they could just have fun and release all of their youthful energy. During the summer and other school breaks, they would be there all day.

Basketball, as a result of their early introduction to the sport in their youth, has continued to play a major role throughout their entire life. Dale II didn't start off playing basketball in junior high and high school because he was a very good drummer and marched in the band starting in the 8th grade. However, once in high school, he started beating rhythms on his desk and not focusing on his schoolwork. So, we made him stop the band. Somehow, the basketball coach must have seen him play during lunch and asked if he could try out. I believe he was in the 10th grade at the time. The coach said to us, "Have you ever seen him play? His reach is phenomenal." My husband and I agreed to let him play on the team and the rest is history. Dale II played the rest of High School and throughout College. Today, he is a High School Math teacher and Assistant Basketball Coach.

Once Dale II started playing basketball, his love and passion for the game has always continued uninterrupted. Daniel on the other hand, played basketball throughout Junior High, High School and also in College. Although he still plays occasionally, he has become more passionate about his career in law enforcement. He currently works as a School Resource Officer for Atlanta Public schools.

Overall, for our entire family, basketball became an integral part of our lives. Starting in high school, both my husband and I began traveling with our sons and their AAU team throughout the Southeastern United States. Then, once they went off to college—Dale earned a full basketball scholarship to LaGrange College and Daniel to Paine College—we were right there in the stands at a majority of their games, both home and away. So, we did a lot of traveling to say the least.

For the most part, because our sons stayed so busy with athletics and other extracurricular activities, we rarely had to worry about discipline issues or even their academics. They knew if they didn't get good grades they wouldn't be playing. The closest I can ever remember either one of them being in any serious kind of trouble is when Dale was probably a senior in high school and Daniel was in the ninth grade. They had gone shopping with two of their friends. Though totally uncharacteristic of them, their two friends decided to shoplift and were caught on camera by mall security.

This didn't make any sense at all, because the young men came from middle class families and had money to buy whatever they needed or wanted. I guess it was just male hormones at work where two male teenagers wanted to test limits just to see if they could get away with it. Fortunately, none of the kids were arrested. I don't even think they were placed on probation.

I was proud and relieved to find out, after I received the call from mall security to come and pick them up, that my sons were not involved in the shoplifting. They just happened to be in the wrong place at the wrong time with friends who chose to make a very poor decision that could have cost them dearly.

This is unlike some of the other horror stories during this period of time in Atlanta in which some of Dale and Daniel's friends had to do real jail time. Totally perplexing once again, these also were young men who came from two-parent homes with great incomes. They just chose to make some poor choices.

I probably can't say it enough, but Dale and Daniel were blessed to not only have their father fully present. Their father was emotionally invested in them. He paid attention to every little detail of their lives and I think that may have been the difference between our boys not veering off and making risky choices that they knew really could have cost them down the line. These are the kinds of conversations their father was constantly having with them: What are the consequences of your choices, your actions, your decisions? With that being said, he wasn't a good father. He was an amazing father!

The Concept of Motherhood

I believe the dictionary defines **Motherhood** as the state or experience of having or raising a child. Giving birth is one aspect of **Motherhood**, and it's not easy. Carrying a baby inside of you for 9 months takes a major toll on your mind, body and spirit. You're tired, nauseated, growing bigger, have swollen feet, etc. Then, during delivery, you will experience excruciating pain and countless emotional highs and lows of, waiting, dilating, water breaking, more pain, more waiting, fully dilated, more pain and so on.

But guess what.... I did it a second time and have no regrets. When I found out I was pregnant with my 2nd son, I felt the same sense of joy and excitement as I did the first time. It's a feeling I can't easily explain. The sense of joy I felt knowing I was going to be a parent was the same feeling I had when my son told me I was going to be a Grandmother.

Motherhood for me was an expression of the love two people have for each other and creating a life to bring into this world. Raising a child is another aspect of Motherhood. Once again, it's not always easy but definitely worth the sacrifice. You, for example, have to reprimand at times and show tough love. This is a major requirement of being a parent. You must be willing to discipline and set boundaries in order for the life that you brought into the world to have a chance of turning out to be productive, well-mannered citizens who can contribute to the world they live in.

How Motherhood Changed My Life

You learn a whole new level of love. Yes, you love your spouse, your mother, your father, your siblings, etc. But that love you have for your child, it's hard to explain. There's an instinct level of self-sacrifice that kicks in. I know, for example, when they were little and became sick or fell down, I felt sick myself. I was willing to do whatever I could to take away their pain.

I think Motherhood also changes your outlook on life. Whereas you might take risks or make some not so great decisions when you're a single person, once you have a child, you have to think about what you're doing, because it's affecting not just you, but your child. Although, when I went into business, I was taking a risk that it could fail, I focused on the upside. I was able to freely go on field trips, volunteer in their school, etc. It afforded me a lot of time to be with my children. By the way, after nearly 30 years of being in business, it hasn't failed yet – "Thank You God!"

Now that my sons are grown and have children of their own, it gives me so much joy to see them raising their little ones. They are both great fathers: taking and picking up their children from daycare; going to the doctor; going to school programs; and, overall, participating in every aspect of their daily lives. I feel like my sons are emulating what they saw in us as parents when they were growing up. This has been a very rewarding feeling for me as a parent to the point that, of all the things I've done in my life, it has made becoming a mother one of my greatest accomplishments.

Lessons on Motherhood

1. When you find out you are pregnant, follow your doctor's regime. Whoever you choose, follow their instructions. Take your vitamins. Don't miss doctor's appointments, etc.

2. As they are growing up, do whatever you can to ensure their good health and overall safety. Again, it's important to take your children to the doctor and to the dentist or regularly scheduled checkups and cleanings. This includes getting their appropriate immunizations.

3. When they begin school, become active. Join the PTA. Volunteer on a committee.

4. Never miss Parent Teacher Conferences. Even if you have to reschedule one-on-one meetings with teachers, this is when you get invaluable information on your children's learning style and habits and their work habits and social skill development.

5. As you children get older, continue to listen to them. Don't just talk, talk, talk nonstop using your authority as a parent to keep them silent. Instead, listen intently and purposefully engage them in mature dialogue. This is a way of preparing them to be adults who know how to communicate with other adults in all situations.

6. When they are going through their challenges, again, listen to them before reacting. Yes, that can be very difficult, but it's important to get the full story first so you can figure out the best way to help them.

7. On a final note, Remember, you are your son or daughters first:

   - Teacher
   - Role-Model
   - Advocate

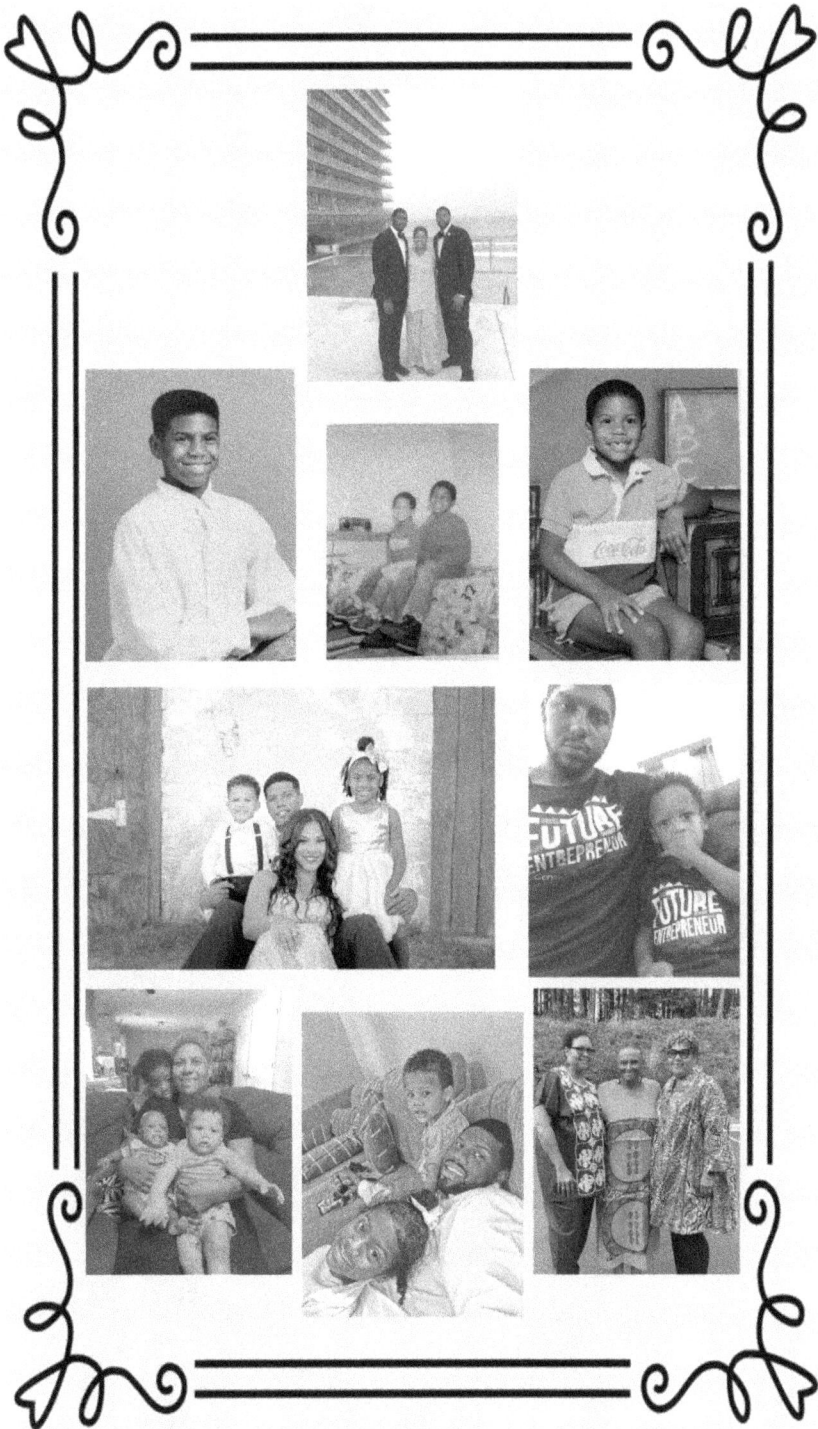
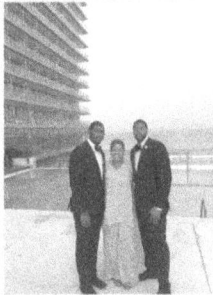
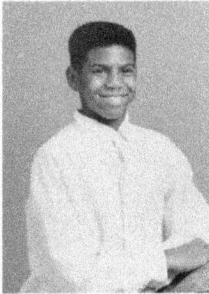
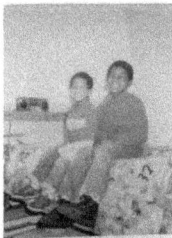
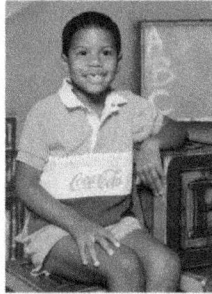
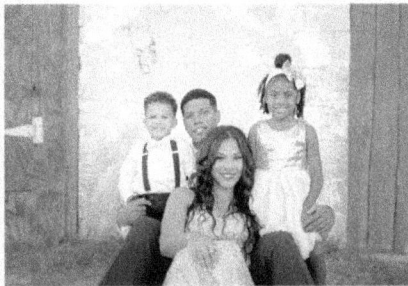
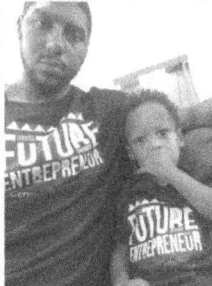
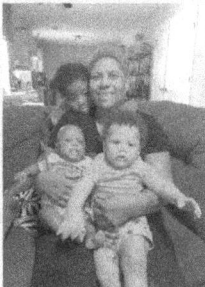
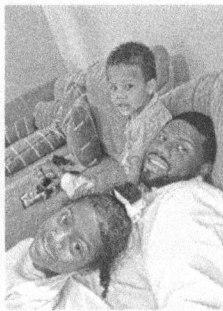
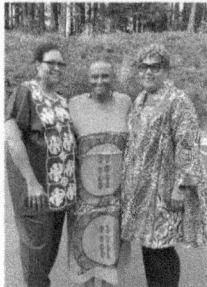

CHAPTER 5
ENTREPRENEURSHIP

Oprah Winfrey is an inspiration to many women around the world. Even more, her stronghold on the world of media is so pervasive that when I think of the word "entrepreneur", without hesitating, Oprah Winfrey's name and image is the first one that pops in my mind. Second place would probably be the husband and wife team of former President Barack and Michelle Obama. Michelle recently released her book, *Becoming* and now it's on Netflix as a documentary. Thirdly, the late Madam C.J. Walker, who was an entrepreneur, a philanthropist and political social activist. She is recorded as the first female self-made millionaire in America. She developed and marketed a line of cosmetics and hair care products for black women. Her documentary was also a mini-series on Netflix.

These are all legendary figures, whom I am sure millions of other Americans have also looked up to and been inspired by. These phenomenal people have made deep impressions in my subconscious mind about what it means to be an entrepreneur. For years, I admired them to such a degree that many of their accomplishments seemed unattainable for a person such as myself. Yet, one day, when I stopped for a moment to put their fame and fortune to the side and was able to just think of them as everyday people who had the courage to follow their dreams and their passions, I realized I have much more in common with them than I originally thought. Just like them, I started with a vision, and with very little money. I, too, was willing to step out on faith in pursuit of making my vision come true. And, here it is nearly 30 years later, V&L Research and Consulting, Inc. (V&L Research) is still in business.

I'd like to give you a little perspective on the significance of this accomplishment—or rather "our" accomplishment, because I have not traveled this road alone. V&L Research would not have been founded, let alone grown as it has, without my business partner Dydra H. Virgil. She's the one who not only planted the seed. Through all these years, she has worked tirelessly to grow and build the company.

Now, getting back to the point I was about to make regarding the significance of our accomplishment of having been in business for nearly 30 years. Did you know that according to an article in Forbes Finance (October 25, 2018) only about half of small businesses survive past the five-year mark (45.5% - 51%)? Beyond that, only one in three small businesses get to the 10-year mark.

V&L Research isn't a million dollar a year company yet. But, we've made millions over its' lifespan thus far. Even more, there are other invaluable ways to measure the success of a business. For one, I take great pride in the fact that once I left Corporate America, I've never had to go back to punching a time clock and working for someone else. So, if, in the end, this will be my claim to fame as an entrepreneur, then I will take it.

Believe it or not, the inspiration to start our business came in a very roundabout way. Our story is not one in which we were losing sleep every night dying to find a way to start our business; there was no burning desire and intense vision to see our business idea come to reality. Rather, our story is totally the opposite. I, in fact, enjoyed working in Corporate America and planned to settle into a great position with a great company and retire.

From my perspective, I stumbled into entrepreneurship. Or, should I say, life gradually steered me in the direction of being an entrepreneur. Because, if I had not moved to Atlanta with my husband and two boys in 1985, it very likely may not have happened at all.

At the time, I was in my late 20s. My husband and I decided to move to Atlanta in search of better career opportunities. We arrived with great excitement and great optimism. However, when I first arrived in Atlanta, the job search was very tough. I applied for position after position with no success. In an effort to try to understand why I wasn't being hired, I began to inquire as to what was missing on my resume or in my experience. To my surprise, the feedback I was getting was that I was overqualified.

As a result of my inability to immediately find employment, it was a very trying time moving to a new city. For an extended period of time, we had to solely depend on my husband's income to support the entire family. I, however, did my best to maintain a positive attitude. Eventually, I did land a job working for a market research company called Peachtree Surveys.

When first hired by Peachtree Surveys, I ran their phone room. After getting acclimated, I later was entrusted with overseeing qualitative research for a number of their clients. In a nutshell, qualitative research "focuses on obtaining data through open-ended and conversational communication. This method is not only about 'what' people think, but also 'why' they think what they think" (https://www.questionpro.com/blog/qualitative-market-research/). While I suspect it probably isn't the kind of work the average person would enjoy doing, for me working in the field of Market Research was highly enjoyable regardless of the task that was asked of me.

I had a good three-year stint at Peachtree Surveys before landing a higher paying job at another market research company called Warner Associates. They offered me a significant pay increase. The icing on the cake was that I would now be working for a black-owned company.

My first day at work felt like a fairy tale. I had lived in a mixed community growing up in Akron. But, to be in a professional, corporate work environment where there's nothing but black people—from the janitors all the way up to the executives and owner of the company—was exhilarating. Well, to be completely honest, there was one non-black employee in the company. His right-hand person and the one who hired me was a Caucasian woman. We still keep in touch to this very day. Matter of fact, over the years, she has worked off and on for V & L Research.

Meeting the owner of the company felt like an honor and a privilege. This was the closest I had ever been to someone so successful in the business world. I was highly impressed by what this black man was able to build and accomplish in the highly competitive market research industry. Remember, this was the late 80s, so, to find a black-owned market research company in such a niche industry was a rarity. I was very excited to say the least.

On an entirely different level, I was ecstatic and grateful to be working in a mostly black environment. The greatest appeal in moving to Atlanta, for my husband and I, in addition to greater career opportunities, was the opportunity to live in a large metropolitan city that was predominantly African-American. And, not just that, but to be surrounded by so many blacks who were living very well... I mean living the middle class and upper middle-class lifestyle.

Both students of Black History, we were well aware of Atlanta's rich history of producing Black Mayors, politicians, countless highly successful entrepreneurs and so on. So, within a few years of moving to Atlanta, to be able to secure a position in my field with such a well-established black-owned company, we were full of confidence that we had made the right decision in packing up from our hometown roots of Akron, Ohio.

The sense of utopia I felt at my new job, unfortunately, did not last long. The owner of the company, whom I initially was so impressed with, all of a sudden turned out to be a totally high-strung, unpredictable and unstable leader. He began to exhibit extreme inconsistencies in his words and in his actions. I witnessed certain decisions he made and certain interactions with other employees, and even clients, that made me shake my head in total disbelief wondering "How in the world did this man build this company to be a multimillion-dollar enterprise????!!!

I will never forget one particular incident in which he had a "meltdown" in the office in front of a handful of employees. He totally flipped out.

We received a request for a proposal on a Monday, and he said it was due on Friday. However, the very next day, on Tuesday, he comes to the office and says, 'Do you have that proposal ready?"

We all looked at each other and said "We're workin' on it... You said it was due by Friday. "

Just like that, in the blink of an eye, the owner went ballistic. He began taking both of his hands, with his arms fully extended out of in front of his body, and brushing them in a broom sweeping motion, from left to right across the desk and knocking everything to the floor. He then went to another desk and repeated the same thing. After a while, he just started picking up things and throwing them.

Never having seen a person have a fit like that, I was scared out of my mind and temporarily froze up. He had this look in his eyes like someone who was possessed.

The feeling of fear and shock brought me to tears. I instinctively ran next door. As he exited out of the office and down the hall, still in a tirade, I could see him from the other office window I was looking out of halfway hiding, yet still looking in disbelief.

The moment was so surreal that off and on for the next 30 minutes I continued to cry uncontrollably. Several co-workers tried to comfort me, as we by then had huddled into a semi-circle in one of the offices. The employees, for the next few hours, tried to console one another and make sense out of what had just happened.

The experience was so traumatic that I don't recall going to work the next day. I, in fact, may have taken a couple of days off before returning. When I did return to work, the memories of what had occurred were not easily erased. The first time I saw the owner of the company walking down the hall it took everything within my power not to shake my head and point my finger at him saying, "You owe me and everyone else an apology."

While I did not have the courage to start looking for a new job, many other employees did. In fact, within a few weeks, my now business partner Dydra found another job at Mercy Medical Center which was part of St. Joseph Health Systems.

Dydra called me one day and asked if I was interested in an Analyst position at the company where she was working. One of her selling points was that I would be reporting to her. Without directly saying it, we both knew what she was trying to convey was that I wouldn't have to worry about any bosses acting crazy. So, I said "Of course I'm interested."

I interviewed and did get the position. As promised, I reported directly to Dydra and we shared an office. She was the Manager of the Strategic Planning Department and I was an Analyst. We were responsible for collecting analytical data on things like surgeries and procedures conducted by doctors throughout the hospital. We also assisted with gathering research and writing reports for the hospital and the entire health system.

There was an immediate supervisor above Dydra who would come in every week or so to review our work. She was Vice President of the Strategic Planning department. To stay organized and keep up with various projects, she loved writing sticky notes. She loved them so much that she would stick them everywhere in our office and on any documents she reviewed.

Overall, this was an enjoyable job with a nice work environment. In addition to being fortunate enough to work with a good friend, everyone in the department generally got along. While management occasionally dumped unrealistic demands on us, it was nothing compared to our last employer.

For a good year, things went along smoothly at my new job. There were no major crises or conflicts. Then, just out of the blue, once Dydra became pregnant and went on maternity leave, the dynamics in the work environment suddenly changed. There wasn't anything in particular that I could put my finger on; it just wasn't the same.

What I do clearly remember, within weeks of Dydra returning from maternity leave was her asking me, "Would you ever want to do this on your own?" I didn't have an immediate answer. But, as her question slowly sunk in, I replied, "Definitely!"

I soon discovered what had prompted her to ask me that question. There was another lady who worked for our company that had already decided to branch out on her own. At some point in her transition, she confided in Dydra that she would need some additional support with contracts getting research and analytics done. And, would we like to do the work on the side?

Of course, we said, "Yes!" Unbelievably, that small side contract turned into several small projects for several months.

This small taste of entrepreneurship wet our appetite. Before I knew it, I was over Dydra's house sitting on the bed in her spare bedroom thinking of company names and logo designs.

Day-by-day our mindset and our focus were becoming more serious and much more intense. We started strategizing where and when to secure office space even if it meant turning one of our spare bedrooms into an office.

Having fully surrendered to the idea of starting our own business and having talked in-depth with our husbands about what this would mean for our families, a new wave of energy and inspiration was pouring through us. I'll never forget the day we came up with the name V&L Research and Consulting. Dydra walked over to the typewriter and just started typing and that's the name she came up with. As soon as I heard it, I knew that was the one.

We weren't even incorporated and didn't have any kind of business license. We, however, were thinking and acting like we were. Even though we were still full-time employees of St. Joseph, we printed business cards and went looking for office space.

It's amazing to think back on that time in my life. For one, we were trying to find our way, trying to navigate the craziness of the corporate world. Secondly, it's a timeline reminder of the bond and close connection that Dydra and I have shared for over 30 years. Her daughter Kayla is now 26 years old.

The first office we looked at was on Memorial Drive in Decatur, a suburb of Atlanta – across the street from the county jail. It was right around 600 square feet. It was small but had just enough room for what we needed. Dydra took the bigger office in the back despite it not having a window, and I took the smaller office in the front. There was a little area in the middle, between the two offices, where we are able to do surveys and recruit for focus groups. Also, there was a reception area and a bathroom. That was it. It was small and compact, but for us it was a huge step and undertaking. I believe the rent was around $600 a month.

Again, we were still at St. Joseph's, working there during the day and then burning the midnight oil. Somehow, not long after we moved into our office, someone at St. Joseph found out that we had a business. We never signed anything that said we could not have a second job or own a business not even in the same industry. Nevertheless, management didn't like it. So, they called us into the office and gave us two choices: Terminate our company or get fired. Without blinking an eye, Dydra and I looked at each other. We, then, turned to executive management, said 'Goodbye' and walked out the door.

We felt such a sense of resolve and determination that we walked out of that St. Joseph building and didn't even go home. We went straight to our office on Memorial Drive.

Where did this level of confidence come from? We knew there was plenty of work out there, more than enough for us to carve out a nice little business where we could make a comfortable living—even though we had not yet built a reputation. However, without question, more than anything, our supreme level of confidence came from the support we received from our husbands.

Long before moving into the office, we had shared with our husbands how passionate we were about the idea of going into business. Neither one of them tried to talk us out of it. When Dydra talked to her husband, he was like, 'Go for it! Then, when I talked to my husband, he gave me 100% support. He was all in as well.

The irony in all of this is that a couple years after resigning from our jobs, both of our husbands started a courier business together. They worked out of our office space. While this was very exciting that all of us were pursuing something entrepreneurial, it also was very scary because no one had a steady, consistent paycheck. Subsequently, it was a very rough financial period in trying to generate enough revenue to support both households.

Somehow, we made it through those tough times and learned many lessons along the way. The reality is that if we never would have started the business there wouldn't be any stories or lessons in entrepreneurship that we could share with others. Once again, without the full support of our husbands, who knows what would have happened? We might never have started any kind of business and just settled and found a way to become content long-term with the idea of working for someone else.

I'll never forget the actual day our employer asked us to shut down our business or resign from St. Joseph. When we got back to the office, a whole new dose of reality hit us. We were like, "What are we going to do now?"

Even though we were still getting projects from our former co-worker from St. Joseph's, that is not the same as having your main 9 to 5 paycheck plus a paycheck from a spouse to add to it.

We didn't sit around long worrying about or feeling afraid that we wouldn't be able to survive. We just put our heads together in thinking about some of the best companies to target for business and immediately started hitting the pavement.

There was a sense of urgency but not panic. We knew it was time to put all our time and energy into marketing and that's what we did. We were determined to make it work, one way or another.

One of the first and best decisions we made was to join different associations. Through these small business associations, we met quite a few people and made some key contacts. We also gained an inside scoop on what was going on in the community and future plans for development. This included learning about new schools they were planning to open. We were perfectly positioned to get the contract to conduct research for the new school.

Not long after that we secured our first big project. It was with the megachurch New Birth Missionary Baptist Church. They, too, were planning to open a school. So, we were contracted to develop an extensive strategic plan for the opening of their school. We interviewed community residents, leaders in the community, and even facilitated focus groups with children and their parents. It was quite an undertaking. To say the least, it was a confidence booster to obtain a contract in the amount of $35,000. More than anything, it helped continue to build forward momentum.

The more we marketed the more we were able to secure contracts, even if they were small projects. This at least allowed us to stay in business. We, for example, would be referred to other asipiring entreprenuers who wanted to start a cake business, or someone who wanted to open up a gym.

There clearly was a tremendous need for the services we were offering. Unfortunately, one of the major obstacles we kept running into was that these weren't clients who had a lot of money to fork out for market research. They needed our services; what we offered was essential to establishing or growing their business. But, they didn't have deep pockets.

So, until we could get in front of enough larger clients with deeper pockets, we had to be very creative with how we did our proposals. Initially, we tried to help everyone. And, we would start out full of passion just so glad to have secured another client. However, we quickly learned that this is not the way to run a business. You must count your potential costs before taking on any project.

We didn't want to turn down anything just because it was so hard to generate business and find new clients. But as you grow, some things are not going to be good for you because you are going to lose money. You must be willing to evaluate and constantly reassess what is working and what isn't working.

Foremost, one of the things I've learned in our nearly thirty years of business is that—because we give the same level of commitment to a $1,000 project as we do to a $100,000 project—going in, we really have to have a clear idea of the number of hours and time it's going to take us to complete the project.

This means that you can't get overly excited just because a potential $100,000 contract is being dangled in front of you. The reality is that a $10,000 project, in the end might yield you a $5,000 to $9,000 profit, where the $100,000 contract may barely break even. Or even worse, you might lose money on the $100,000 project because there's no cap on the demands and requests from the client.

Therefore, if the numbers don't make sense, you have to be willing to walk away from a potential project. In removing the emotion from how you're viewing the potential contract, you have to be willing to accept that you can't help everyone.

Even though we were still learning on the fly how to make better, sound financial decisions in running a business, the good thing is that we were growing. The amount and type of projects we were taking on required us to start considering finding more office space, one where we could have our own facility for conducting focus groups. Whenever we moderated focus groups, we were renting other facilities for the day which was an additional expense.

Then, one day, someone suggested we move into an office space nearby where another research company was in the process of terminating their lease and moving out. We immediately drove down the street to look at the facility, and sure enough, it had exactly what we needed. So, we moved in and took over their lease.

A lot of great things were happening. Yet, it all seemed to be happening so fast that at times I wondered how I was going to keep up. How was I going to stay on top of everything without going out of my mind?

Another significant thing that was occurring was that we really became very disciplined in our marketing efforts. When funds were low, we bartered with one lady that Dydra had met. This Marketing Specialist updated our logo and gave us some great ideas for marketing. We also began to use a friend of mine named Charlotte who had a background in communications. She was so creative that she came up with a full campaign for the grand opening of our new office.

Moving into the new facility took our company to an entirely new level with how we were perceived by potential and current clients and with how we conducted business. Maximizing the ample space, we now occupied, there were a number of things we now could do in-house. At the top of the list was being able to rent out space to other companies who needed a research facility to conduct their focus group projects. In addition to now having a focus room, we did taste-testing and even had requests from other companies to utilize our telephone room.

Despite the creative things we did to generate additional revenue, we still were drowning in overhead costs. The expenses associated with maintaining a much larger office space were very costly. There were copy machines, land line phones with answering machines, additional staff such as a receptionist, administrative assistants and even an office manager.

There also were other impromptu adjustments we had to make on the fly which tested our ability to be flexible and persevere. On one occasion, due to a thunderstorm, the lights went out while conducting a focus group. I knew the bill had been paid. So, I knew that our lights had not been cut off. Thank God we had candles in the office! Because of this, I was able to resume and complete the focus group by candlelight.

On a few other occasions when the power went out, we weren't able to record the interviews we were conducting. So, someone had to jump in and start taking notes. Back then, there weren't any laptops. There were only desktop computers. Quickly learning from these highly stressful occurrences, we started using battery-operated recorders as backups.

Overall, despite the constant challenges we were confronted with, we seemed to find a way to overcome every single one of them. In fact, we continued to steadily grow. One example of this was our decision to move again. This time it wasn't solely due to growth. The area in which our office was located was starting to change and as a result fewer people wanted to come to our area to do research. Thinking ahead, we felt it was best to be proactive and not wait to make the move.

We moved into a larger facility that was near a mall. So, it was a high traffic area. The move was totally different from the others. This time we built out, meaning, our office spaces and facility were built from scratch. We didn't just buy the furniture. We literally designed the rooms which was a very exciting experience for us. It also made us feel very proud and important to have our company name on the outside of the building.

Five years into business, and then ten years, we had found our niche. We started specializing in providing a full range of market research services targeting the African-American and Hispanic population. While we had done all types of research, including specifically for the elderly, affluent and low to moderate income consumers, we were discovering that services specifically for the African-American and Hispanic population had become our bread and butter; or, at least that it could be. Because of the long-term need and our experience and expertise in this area, we felt we should focus most of our attention on going after these kinds of contracts. That turned out to be a great decision for the short-term and the long-term.

Even though we were steadily growing, we had not yet learned how to build up and maintain a large cash reserve. Thus, there was a constant juggling of bills and debt. In fact, on multiple occasions, without the loans that we secured based on invoices that were scheduled to be paid in the next 30, 60, or 90 days, we wouldn't have been able to meet payroll or even avoid getting evicted from our office space.

These loans were a lifesaver, but they were not easy to pay off. Once payment of an invoice came in from one of our clients, we not only had to give that money right back to the lender. We also had to make payment for the interest that had accrued on the loan.

Surprisingly, getting a loan was not a problem at all because we were generating steady income, and they didn't require much paperwork to process the loan. There were just a few papers to sign. The hard part was keeping up with all the bill payment due dates including the $2,000 to $3,000 a month office rent. In short, we were constantly robbing Peter to pay Paul.

The running joke in the office was that I was the "Queen" of the payment plan. I became masterful at calling creditors and bill collectors to set up payment arrangements that were much more manageable for us. My approach was to focus on getting them to agree to allow us to pay half of what was due or even a third.

Getting these revised payment terms was critical because negotiating them down to the lowest monthly payment amount possible gave us breathing room to juggle paying our other monthly recurring expenses and debts to creditors. This included paying a number of employees and contractors we had coming to work for us. This meant making payroll every two weeks for several employees at that time.

In the end, we finally said to ourselves that trying to pay ourselves a decent salary, having full-time staff and contractors and a large office space was too much. It had been a few years of going through the dance of juggling our finances and constantly trying to dig ourselves out of a hole. Even though we should have made drastic changes much sooner, the truth is that we weren't truly ready to make real financial change and more sound financial decisions until we found ourselves in court. We were in court after having fallen several months behind in paying our office rent. This was around 2005/2006.

Being taken to court was the major tipping point when we finally woke up and said "What are we doing? Some of the decisions we are making gotta' change." We realized if we didn't learn to practice better financial management habits we may reach a point where we could lose our business and have to file bankruptcy.

Following the court proceedings, we paid back some of the rent. More importantly, we decided it was time to let the office space go. From that point on, Dydra started working out of her house, and I started working out of mine. Again, that was around 2005/2006, and we have worked from our homes ever since. Even when things were going great financially, just as a best practice to make sure we never pile up too much overhead, we resisted the temptation to lease office space again. We just find that it makes more economic sense to work from our homes. This ensures that we will always have a cushion and wiggle room whenever there's a lull in securing new clients or being paid on time by current clients.

Amazingly, I discovered that I didn't miss having the office as much as I thought I would. Probably, because we already had great office spaces in the past, it wasn't as much of a blow to my ego as I had anticipated. In becoming a more seasoned entrepreneur, I was more comfortable with focusing on the bottom line and more motivated to have something tangible to show for all our hard work.

Without question, we should have made a number of financial changes much sooner. Even from looking at the monthly, quarterly and yearly profits and losses of our business, the writing was on the wall that we needed to eliminate some liabilities. But we were too emotionally invested in keeping things the way they were. In other words, we had become content with just keeping the doors to our business open and not having to return to a 9 to 5. This was combined with the fact that things were happening way too fast. We were doing back-to-back focus groups, traveling a lot and never made it the highest priority to maximize how we managed our finances. We had become accustomed to "surviving" as a mindset and never really believing or understanding what it would take to transition our mindset and our actions to that of a "thriving" business.

It's not like we didn't have someone prepare our annual returns and also make sure we paid our quarterly taxes on time. We just didn't have the right mindset or fully understand the importance of being highly disciplined in sitting down at least once a month for in-depth conversations as a team about our financial picture and then developing a clear plan of what adjustments needed to be made in order to achieve our short-term and long-term goals as a business.

However, once we let go of the office space, this all started to change. For one, it allowed us to sleep better at night because it was one less major bill we had to worry about. Secondly, we were finally learning to measure the true wealth and assets of our business not just by how much revenue we were generating. We began measuring it by the actual net profit we were making—after all company expenses were paid, and how the actual net worth of our company was growing from year to year.

It's amazing how, 30 years later, it's so much easier to have an office presence without taking on the high overhead. There are several places now that will rent office space to you on an as-needed basis. In addition to getting a business address, they have other add-on services like letting you know when you receive mail. So now, we have an Atlanta office address on our business cards for a nominal monthly fee. If we need to meet with clients, we can reserve a conference room for an additional small fee.

The reality is that the annual revenue of V&L Research and Consulting has greatly fluctuated from year to year. Some years we've made $200,000. Other years we've made $600,000. For more than a decade, we had never developed a roadmap for our business. Now, we do. We have written goals as well as regularly scheduled meetings, including an annual meeting where we review our goals and financials.

The entrepreneur I am today is nothing like the entrepreneur I was thirty years ago. While the passion and love for what I do is still there, I have a sense of purpose on how I'm approaching the growth and wealth building of our business. This more seasoned entrepreneurial approach to running our business has made the journey much more rewarding, possibly just as rewarding as being the co-owner of a company in which I can proudly say, "30 years later, I left my 9 to 5 job and never looked back."

Lessons on Entrepreneurship

1. **Always Market Yourself even when you're working on current projects.** This is one of the biggest challenges of small businesses, because you typically don't have enough manpower to fully service the projects you're working on, and keep your clients happy, while actively looking for new business. Being a small business owner, by itself, generally means that you must be very skilled and accustomed to wearing many hats at one time. At the same time, the stages of growth that a company goes through requires that additional staffing be put in place. When we fail to do this, it stifles and stunts the growth of a company.

2. **Setting Goals.** We have set a goal for at least $30,000 per month in proposals. When we finally hit this goal for the very first time, it took several months to reach it. Ever since then, we have not always hit this goal. But as I've learned over the years, if you're going to grow your business, you always have to have a goal to strive for.

3. **Work Smarter and Not Harder.** This is particularly significant because remember what I said earlier in the chapter. We give the same level of commitment to a $10,000 project as we do to a $100,000 project. Before taking on a project, we learned the hard way that you have to carefully count the costs. In other words, calculate what, in the end, will be your real profit. Don't get overly anxious because a potential client is dangling $100,000 in front of you. If you are only going to make $5,000 or just break even, then you may be better off walking away.

4. **Cash Flow and Cash Reserves are essential.** Set a Budget, because all marketing is not free. You've got to be willing to spend money to make money. At the same time, it's important to have Accountability with the Budget you set. Work hand-in-hand with your bookkeeper and/or accountant. Meet with them in-person or by phone at least quarterly, preferably monthly.

5. **Developing and Executing your Business Plan and/or Set Goals.** Many people have heard the term "business plan" but have never actually written one for their business. Believe it or not, we didn't write our first business plan until we had been in business for five years. However, it was necessary for the growth of our company. Have you ever heard the phrase, "Plan your Work and Work your Plan?" It's true, it works.

   It's pretty amazing to think that we survived the threshold of the first few years of being in business, when most businesses fail, despite not having a business plan. While we were fortunate that our business got off to a good start, how much longer could our trajectory of steady growth continued on before we hit a brick wall if only we had first developed a business plan; if we had some kind of roadmap and guideposts to refer back to?

6. **"You can't be everything to all people."** In other words, "You can't help everybody." It's taken us several years, but now that we've found our niche, we focus on what we do best. That is, we're really good at hard-to-reach populations (low income, wealthy, senior populations, etc.). So, knowing and accepting

this, these are the types of proposals we spend the bulk of our time and energy on.

7. **TEAMWORK and COMMUNICATION**. "Working for yourself doesn't necessarily mean working by yourself." Even when you're working by yourself, you still need help from others. Everyone is not an expert on everything. You need to surround yourself with people that have expertise or strengths in your areas of weakness.

   You might already know what you want but don't know how to get there. So, you have to be open to reaching out to others and asking for help. For example, you might need a "Strategist. And, if you can't afford something you really need, be creative in bartering to offer something of value in exchange.

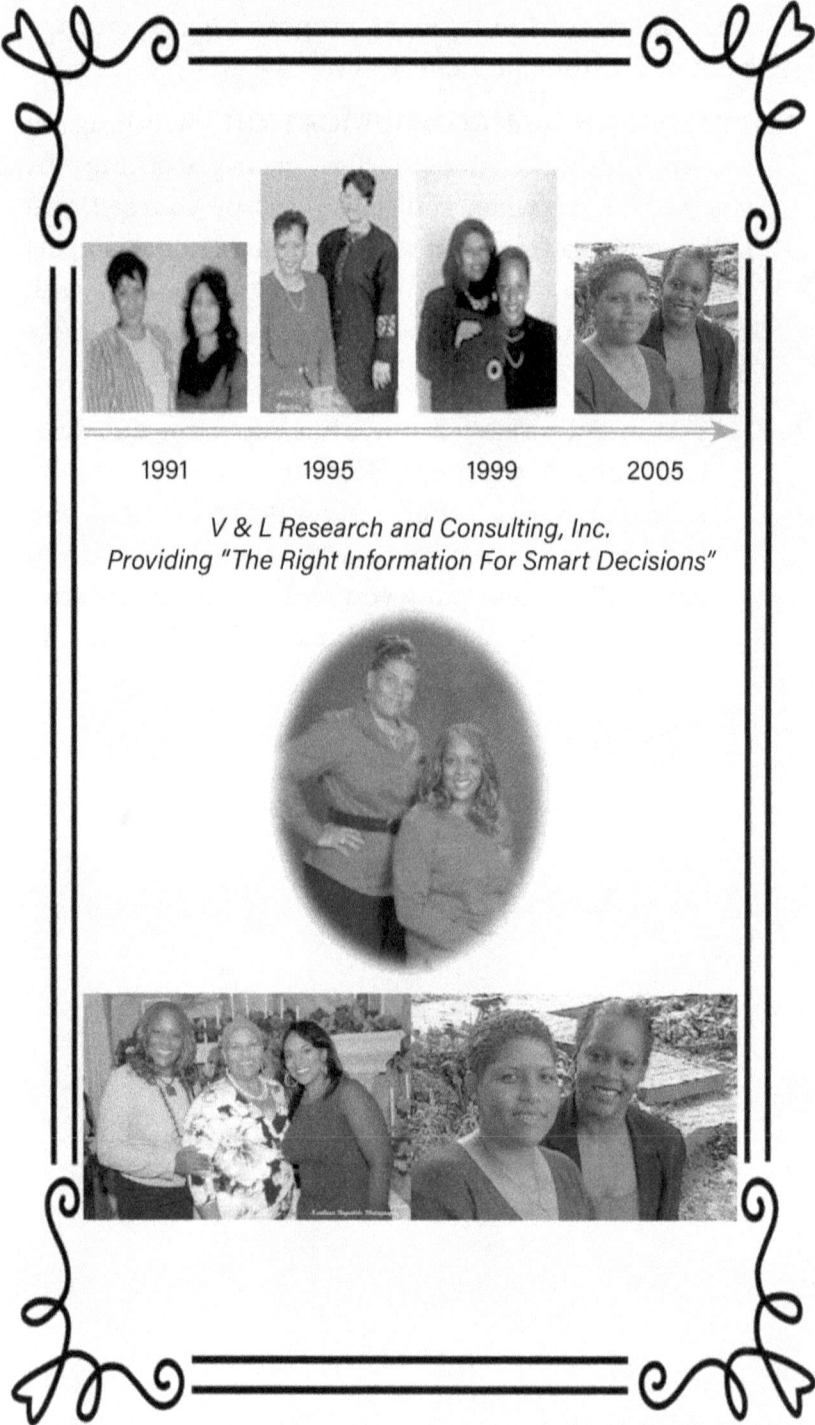

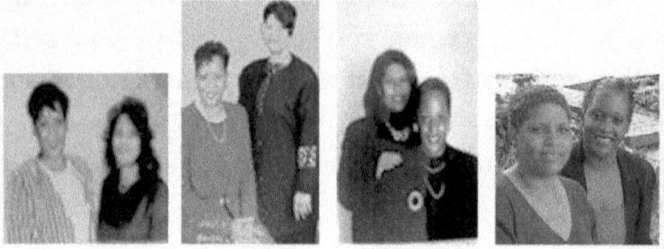

1991   1995   1999   2005

V & L Research and Consulting, Inc.
Providing "The Right Information For Smart Decisions"

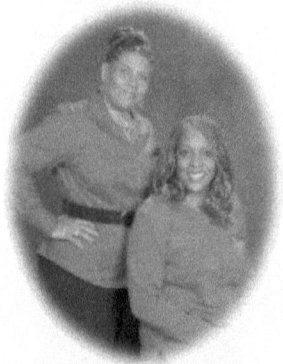

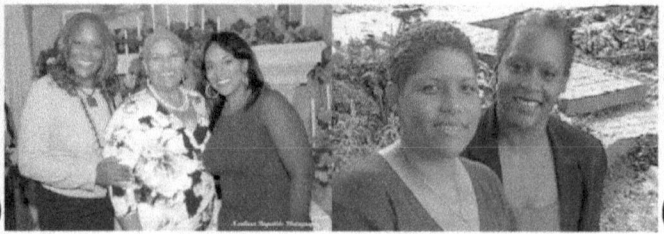

CHAPTER 6
DIVORCE

Til' Death do us part

I thought til' death do us part.
but, he was thinking somethin' else.

I was happy,
But, he wasn't.

How could I have known that he was that unhappy....
unhappy enough to leave a 30-year marriage???

Or, maybe it wasn't a marriage at all?
Maybe we were just sleeping in the same bed
for many years...
never fully sharing the same dream.

Just so totally unbelievable
to think and believe
that for so many years
you're on this journey together,
and that everything is good.

Well,
I guess it wasn't..........

It must not have been good
for a pretty long damn time....
because I woke up from the illusion
I was living in.
I woke up to feeling
the throbbing pain
of being punched in the gut.

I woke up to the harshest dose
of reality:
that it was time to move on
from a marriage of more than 30 years.

That it was time
to deal with the Aftermath from:
The people who are hurt!
The people who are angry!
The people who are equally confused

and searching for answers —
after seeing us for so many years
"seemingly" so Happy,"
"seemingly" Unified as an Unbreakable Team!!!

Now,
beginning the process of
Finding a new church home.
Finding new friends.

I must find a new path
to a new life...

This is the Pain
and Anguish
of Divorce.

- - - - - - - - - -

My primary goal in writing this book was not just to tell my life story. It was to have a heart-to-heart conversation with women of all races and all colors. I wanted to have a conversation about life, love, pursuing your dreams and overcoming hardships. Well, getting a divorce after 30 years of marriage was one of the most painful and heart-wrenching challenges I've had to overcome in my life. So, in the process of writing this book, this was the chapter I dreaded the most.

Even though I knew it was one of the most pertinent conversations I needed to have with my readers, I needed to mentally and emotionally prepare myself to relive the very painful memories of the relationship coming to an end. I needed to prepare myself to revisit the anguish I experienced when a relationship I once thought would last forever, unimaginably came crashing to an end.

For me, hearing the words, "I want a divorce," was worse than the doctor saying, "You have breast cancer."

While Cancer attacked my physical body, Divorce attacked my soul. This is because Marriage is not just a physical connection. It's a soul connection. So, a part of me died when I lost my Marriage. And, I had to find a way to reclaim that lost part of myself.

What made the divorce even more difficult to cope with was the fact that I didn't see it coming. I felt like I was blindsided. Or, maybe I was a victim of my own unwillingness to deal with the truth and the reality that had been right in front of me for some time: for months and possibly even years.

Looking back on it, I guess that deep down I knew something wasn't right. I knew something had been altered in the chemistry between the two of us, but I didn't have the remedy or cure for restoring the magic in our marriage.

My life was going 90 miles an hour, as I was constantly traveling for business. So, maybe I should have put more weight on the fact that he had started to spend significantly more time on his phone and on the computer than spending quality time as a couple. But, once again, the train of life was going 90 miles an hour, and I was more focused on trying to keep up with the speed of my life rather than taking my life by the reins and forcing it to slow down.

Maybe I had become too content with the assumption that, after thirty years of marriage, we were safe; we were secure enough to weather any challenges; we were on the same page with our future life goals despite how fast our lives were moving: that this could never be the downfall of our marriage.

When? Where? And, How? These are the three questions I repeatedly asked myself as I obsessively looked back in time, trying to find the chink in our marital armor.

My best guess would be that major cracks started to form in our marriage sometime in 2009. It was in 2009 that my business partner and I secured one of our most lucrative contracts to date. The contract was with American Family Insurance. They were doing a study on African-American consumers.

Leading up to landing this contract, there was quite an extensive proposal bidding process. All the travel with my job, combined with constantly having to be on the grind to find new business, kept me away from family quite a bit. And, during this period of time is when I started to feel something wasn't quite right in our marriage. Ironically, at the very end of 2009, he and I headed to Los Angeles to spend the week. We had a really good time on our trip.

Upon returning home, I reenlisted in Weight Watchers as part of my New Year's Resolution. Keeping my weight down had been a major tug of war for several years, and I felt that it had finally taken a toll on him. I must give him credit though. For a number of years, he had been extremely supportive of my efforts to lose weight and keep it off. He was so supportive that he joined Weight Watchers with me. And, he never said anything negative to me about my weight. I just think, after a number of years and countless attempts to tackle this problem once and for all, he ran out of energy. More than anything, I think he became disappointed in me and my inability to manage my weight. For him, as a relatively fit person himself, my belief is that he began to find me less attractive because of it.

In February 2010, the emotional distance between us became even more apparent. This was the first time that I verbalized my concern to him. Previously, I assumed it was just a phase we were going through, and that it would pass. But now, I knew and was starting to accept the fact that we were clearly in the danger zone. So, I asked him, "Is everything okay?" He confidently responded, "Sure, everything is fine."

March 2010, I planned a birthday bash at our house for our youngest son who was turning 25. It turned out to be a Birthday Bash for anyone born in the month of March. So that included him, our oldest son and other family and friends who were born in the month of March. It was well attended and such a great evening that weeks and months later people were still talking about how amazing the party was.

March also was the month that my business partner and I were officially awarded the American Family Insurance contract. Securing the $250,000 contract was an exhilarating feeling! Yet, it was just a few weeks later, if not days, that the tragedy of our divorce struck. That's when my husband said the unthinkable, "I WANT A DIVORCE!!!

His words were spoken in a soft voice tone much like we were having a normal conversation. Immediately, however, I felt the weight of his words. They were so heavy that they felt as though someone had ripped my heart out, which caused me to drop to my knees sinking to the floor. The moment, filled with a rush of emotion, fully overwhelmed me much like answering the phone to be told that a loved one had just DIED .

The devastating news was delivered to me as he sat at his desk in his office. We had been looking over our budget and some of the upcoming bills that soon would be due. That's when he turned to me, looked up as I was standing beside him, and said, "I WANT A DIVORCE!"

It was an out-of-body experience where, on some audible level, I did hear what he said. Yet, on another level, or in another realm, I really didn't hear a single word.

Feeling as though someone had just kicked me in my stomach while ripping out my heart, my spirit temporarily left my body. I was no longer conscious of this physical reality. The moment had instantly produced deep moans of anguish in which I was compelled to cry out, "NO!!! NO!!! NO!!!"

Then, a flood of intimate memories between him and I rushed through my mind: I met him at the age of 9; he asked me for my number at the age of 14; we went on our first date at age 16; we went to the high school prom; we got married at age 21; we had our children at age 24 and age 27.

Now that the kids are gone, this was supposed to be our time to settle in with each other, our time to connect and bond on a whole new level. Instead, we were tearing apart more than thirty years of marriage. The opportunity to continue to work on mending the relationship was taken off the table. You, instead, had already come to peace with your decision to build a whole new life with someone else.

How could this be happening to me?

How could my life be crumbling and falling apart like this?

Yes. We were struggling with money, just like we had many times before. But we always found a way out. Right in front of us, my getting the new big contract was another example of it. Somehow, this just wasn't enough for him to stay. It couldn't mend whatever wounds or damage had already been done to him as a man, and as my husband.

I also clearly remember, after he asked for a divorce, that in May 2010, he decided to go on a bike trip out west for a couple of weeks with one of his brothers. I guess he felt it would help him clear his head. Or possibly, it was just part of his new mission to find personal happiness—a long unfulfilled item on his bucket list.

I wasn't so bitter and angry that I resented him going on his trip. I just was perplexed as to why he felt now was the time for something like this. Despite having so many unanswered questions about why he had decided to end our marriage and attempt to remove items from his bucket list, I remained cordial and non-adversarial during the transition. In an effort to hold on to our marriage or at least in trying to maintain our lifelong friendship, I remained highly supportive of him by doing things like going with him and his brother to purchase different items they needed for their trip.

Unfortunately, because of a motorcycle accident that occurred during their trip, it was abruptly cut short. More significantly, during the short period of time that they were on the road, I received a major revelation. I discovered he was talking to another woman. While he still would call me from the road to check-in, he was also calling the other woman at the same time.

When I confronted him about this other woman, he stood his ground in arguing that he was not leaving me because of her. He point blank said, "I would have left you anyway!"

In addition to there being another woman who now was holding his attention, I couldn't stop thinking or believing that the number one reason he was leaving me was because of my weight. Internally, psychologically, there was a tape playing over and over in my head saying, "YOU'RE TOO FAT!" YOU'RE TOO FAT!" So, I became obsessed with getting the weight off.

One day, while walking in a park, I noticed this very fit guy helping a lady do some exercise drills. I walked up to him and asked if he was a trainer. He said, "Yes." And, just like that, I hired him to start training me.

Losing weight, with the goal of regaining my amazing figure, became a major focal point and emotional and physical outlet to help me deal with my heartbreak. It had been several weeks since my husband told me he wanted a divorce. Yet, I still had not reached out to anyone for emotional support. I purposely was hiding from everyone. I was just too embarrassed.

When I finally reached the point where I just couldn't hold it in any longer, the person I finally decided to confide in was a very good friend of mine. I possibly picked her because we used to work out together. After telling her what was going on, I felt a little better.

To my surprise, a few days later, I found out that, without asking my permission, she called my husband to question him about the reasons for him wanting to get a divorce. I was furious!!! My conversation between the two of us was supposed to be totally confidential.

She made matters worse by asking me, "Have you talked to him from his perspective?"

How unbelievable of her to ask me this and to reach out to him without my permission. I felt embarrassed as well as deeply hurt by her doing this. To be more honest, I felt like a fool for having selected her as the sole person to confide in.

Now that the cat was out of the bag, more and more family members started to talk to each of us. As expected, though unwanted, they tried to interject their opinions on what caused the downfall of our marriage and what was needed to save it. Yet, none of them were being very helpful. They mostly made matters worse by telling me things that sounded more and more confusing than what I had already heard or been told.

I already knew or had heard his reasons for wanting a divorce. At the top of the list was his feeling like he was in my shadow — which I still have a hard time interpreting. Secondly, he said he wasn't "happy" anymore; that I was a good wife and an excellent mother, but he wasn't "happy".

One of the most bizarre things that one of my relatives said to me after talking to him was, "What if you came home and found him in the garage with his brains blown out?' I was like 'What are you talking about!?!?! Is it really that bad?' It took me a long time to process that statement. Even worse, hearing this from my relative made me wrestle with and try to figure out even more what the hell my husband meant by, "I'm not HAPPY!?!?"

To me, happiness is what you make it, especially in a relationship. If you're not happy in a relationship, the two people should sit down to talk about what's not making them happy so that they can try to fix it. They can try to make adjustments.

Unfortunately, I was never given the opportunity to make any adjustments. I was never given the opportunity to try and fix our marriage. One day, I was just told that it's over: "I'm done. I'm moving on."

After thirty years of marriage, I at least thought I was owed an opportunity to make things right. Particularly knowing that I was 100% invested in the marriage, why couldn't I have been given this opportunity?

The more I pressed my husband for answers to these questions the more he just expressed that it was not an easy decision. That he literally had been walking around Stone Mountain Park crying fearing the pain and devastation the news would cause me. That he tried to rehearse the right words to say, but just didn't know how to tell me.

This explanation infuriated me even more now that I had the additional information of him having already been talking to another woman. This put a totally different spin on the reasons for our breakup. I now had a totally different perspective of his wanting to leave the relationship. There was another outside influence and future prospect that was awaiting his departure from our marriage. Again, he kept telling me I didn't leave you for another woman. How ironic? It's the same woman he broke up with me to date when we were in High School.

Maybe I was overthinking things or just thinking too highly of myself. But, time and time again, I just kept wondering, "If it wasn't for the other woman, would he have stayed and at least tried to work things out?" "Would he have told me what all of his issues and concerns were before deciding that it just wasn't going to work; that he just couldn't find "happiness" in our marriage any longer?"

The reality, however, was that he was far, far ahead of me in deciding to get a divorce. He had planned it. So, it really wasn't hard for him to say he wanted a divorce because he was already there. He had already left the building without going to marital counseling of any kind. I was the one who had to try and play catch-up. This was an emotional and psychological process that took months, really a few years for me to accomplish.

Fast forward to just a few weeks later when I was faced with another test. All on the same day, it was Mother's Day and our oldest son's fiancé' was graduating from college in South Carolina. My husband and I traveled together to the graduation, but I was an emotional wreck. It really would have been best for me to have stayed home. I was so sick inside that his brother tried to console me by giving me scriptures to read. Although they were very helpful, I still continued to fall apart.

After the graduation ceremony, I spent more time in the bathroom crying than I did enjoying time with family. Everyone was trying to figure out what was going on. What was wrong with me? My mom was there, and both of the graduate's parents were there.

I just kept trying to fake it to make it by pretending that everything was okay. In my mind, I had a reputation to uphold of having the perfect relationship, of being the perfect couple. So, I chose to fake marriage rather than just let everyone know the truth of what I was dealing with. This had to have been the worst Mother's Day of my life.

A couple months later, July 2010, at my dad's family reunion in Rome, Georgia, I continued with the charade by attending the reunion instead of just staying home. People could tell something was wrong with me. It was that obvious. My mother later said that she thought I was going through menopause.

During this same family reunion, this is when he shared with me that he was planning to move to Chicago. It came to me in a roundabout way. He didn't sit me down to specifically tell me that this is what he was planning to do. It was when I asked him to take me to the airport to catch a flight for a business trip that he said he couldn't take me. The reason was because he was leaving town for a job interview in Chicago.

I had already been overwhelmed by the news of him wanting a divorce. This just added to the feelings of disbelief and bewilderment that had slowly but steadily been strangling and suffocating me over the last few months in my efforts to try to cope and function in my daily life. The pain and anguish intensified when I heard such ugly words come out of his mouth, "I don't desire you anymore!"

I was like, "OH MY GOD!!! Has it really gotten that bad? What have I done to deserve this???"

More than ever before, I knew this was really the end of our marriage. I knew that there would be no turning back for him. He was full steam ahead in executing his plan for his new future (without me).

Divorce was no longer an illusion. It was imminent. The only question now was how and when. He was so determined to get a divorce that he even threw out the idea of filing for divorce online instead of sitting down with lawyers. I adamantly refused. In the end, we did go see an attorney. A member from our church, who was an attorney, offered to draw up the paperwork for free. So, we scheduled an appointment.

On the day of the appointment, he and I rode together which I soon discovered was a major mistake. Too many emotions were being triggered by the impending end of our marriage. With each step we took headed up the stairwell to our attorney's office, I more and more could feel a tidal wave of emotions welling up inside of me. Before we could reach the top of the stairs, I broke down crying and ran to the ladies room to try and gather myself. Once inside of the attorney's office, seated with my arms folded across the other, I remained quiet throughout the entire meeting.

The attorney shuffled several papers. She, then, organized them in a neat pile and slid them to the front of her desk as if to invite us to review them. Just then, she looked both of us directly in the eye and said, "Are you sure about this?"

He replied first, "Yes."

I just looked at him without ever replying to the attorney. He never look back at me. He just turned his head and looked out the window.

The attorney, then, directed us to go to a notary. We went to Georgia Federal Credit Union near LaVista Road.

In the notary's office, we were greeted by a middle-aged African-American woman who was very friendly and lighthearted. I think she could sense the mood and heaviness of emotion that was in the air. When she was finally ready for us to sign, she did the exact same thing our attorney had done less than an hour earlier. She asked us, "Are you sure about this?"

My husband, once again, in a tone and mannerism that was full of confidence said, "Yes."

I, on the other hand, could not utter a word. Bursting into tears, I told my husband I would wait for him in the Tahoe. After signing the papers, I quickly stood up and left the room.

He Officially Moves Out of The House

Before he left in August 2010, very close friends (Sunserai Bell and Kathy Ragland) took me on a trip to Gatlinburg, Tennessee. Amazingly, since our first trip together, we've gone on countless other trips: Costa Rica; Bahama's; Las Vegas for New Year's Eve; New York City; Florida; and this past January 2020 the Australian Open. On the way back from the trip, I called him and asked about my health insurance. I wanted to confirm that, even though we were getting a divorce, I would still be covered under his insurance. He did not hesitate in replying, "How about you get your own?"

The reality is that, as an entrepreneur, I had been covered by the health insurance plan of my husband's employer for years. This would be a new expense I would have to find a way to cover in addition to all the other expenses I now would be assuming sole responsibility for. The new contract with American Family Insurance could not yet be counted as real income for another 30 to 60 days. So, basically, we were broke.

Despite our current financial challenges, my husband still found a way to execute his plan. On August 24, 2010, he officially moved out the house. Given how tight money was for us as a couple, it made me wonder how in the world he was able to come up with the money to move all the way to Chicago?

Every single item that belonged to him was completely removed. He left no traces of his prior existence in our home except for some family photos and various handyman work that he built or repaired throughout the years.

Fortunately, some friends, having witnessed my frequent moments of emotional fragility over the last few months, anticipated this day would be one of the hardest, if not the hardest for me. So, they came and took me away. They insisted I not be anywhere near the house on the day he officially moved out.

Sure enough, when I returned home it was as if the house had been robbed. Even though the house was still filled with furniture, there was just a pervasive feeling of emptiness, sadness and grief. The grief then turned to anger as I pounded on the kitchen table and finally cried myself to sleep on the living room sofa.

Being in that house by myself, the days were very long and lonely. Unable to fully heal and move on, I longed for a sense of closure. I tried to be strong and work through this painful ordeal on my own, but it was just too much to bear. An instinctive part of me literally called out for my mother. I picked up the phone, crying in tears saying, "I need mommy!!!"

One month later, September 2010, my Mom came to live with me. I remember my youngest son Daniel driving with me to Akron, Ohio Labor Day weekend to move her to Georgia.

Though my husband had filed for divorce in 2010, it wasn't final until July 2011, nearly a year after he filed the paperwork. To finalize our divorce, we were required to appear in court in front of a judge. It then would be official.

The day of our court hearing was like a scene out of a movie. Rather than feeling like a court appearance, it felt like I was on trial. I mean it was a weird feeling to be sitting in a room with so many other couples who were also getting a divorce. It was like one big performance where each act is called to the stage, one at a time, to perform in front of a ready-made audience.

Because there wasn't much argument about splitting our property and other assets, the proceedings were short and quick. He had already decided to give me the house. To my total amazement, he didn't ask for any equity or financial compensation of any kind. He just wanted out of the marriage. He wanted to be free to move on with his life.

The judge, however, was not satisfied with just leaving it at that. She sharply commented to him, "If she defaults on the loan for the house, you are still liable." Therefore, there was an added stipulation that after two years I would have to put the house solely in my name.

Once that was added to the record, the judge then turned to me and asked, "Do you want a divorce?" I stared back at him and said, "No. But I don't want anybody who doesn't want me!"

You could hear people in the courtroom going, "Ooooh" and "Ahhh...."

The judge then turned to him and asked the same question. He seemingly and effortlessly, just as the many times before, said, "Yes."

Lessons on Divorce

1. How ironic that, as I finish writing this chapter of the book on "Divorce," I look at the calendar and realize it's occurring in the same month as when my ex-husband asked me for a divorce (the month of March). It's the same month as when I got the big business contract and the same month as when we celebrated a huge family milestone. Even more, while dictating a sentence in the chapter to my co-writer, it also suddenly hit me like a ton of bricks that the actual date in which we're working on this chapter for the first time is the birthday of my first husband. Today is March 13th, 2018 and it's his 61st birthday. WOW!!! How synchronistic or ironic?

   > For me, while years removed from the physical relationship with my first husband, the irony of writing about the finalization of our divorce on the same day as his birthday is a clear reminder that I do not need to disown or attempt to negate the significance of my more than 50-year relationship with him. While it ended on a sour note, and there were a number of years in the early stages of our relationship that brought me great pain and anguish, in the end, it wasn't all bad. And, that's what I need to focus on. **It was time to stop being the Victim and be the Victor!**

2. More importantly, in moving forward, as part of the process of healing and forgiveness, **I need to focus on all the good that existed and occurred in our relationship. And, I also need to take responsibility for what I helped create in the relationship over the years, the good and the bad.** We raised a family and

built a home. We truly did build a home, not in the physical sense: hundreds if not thousands of people experienced our home as a place not just for entertainment and social gatherings, but as a respite, and as a place for spiritual counsel.

3. So, just as there has been tremendous pain in our relationship. There also has been tremendous beauty. And, in walking through my conversation today with my co-author, I was able to see how the beauty and pain of our relationship symbolizes the level of connection that will forever exist between my first husband and me.

> By adopting this new perspective of our relationship, I no longer need to hate him or hate that I ever made the decision to marry him. I need to celebrate and cherish the love that did exist between us for many years. I need to forgive him and more importantly forgive myself for the part I played in helping create the long-term life experiences that were deeply painful. This is the only way that I could truly be free of my anguish. **This is the only way that I could be free to move on with my life.**

Additional Lessons on Divorce

Taking on this new perspective—even in the midst of grieving and working through feelings of anger—for spouses to move on if you haven't, there are several things you can do. Try writing a letter or talking to those who have hurt or abandoned you. You need to find a release. For me, I wrote him a letter and I had a conversation with her (my ex-husbands new girlfriend). If you are going to be around people who hurt you and you want to get closure, you must find a way to release that negativity if truly are going to heal and find happiness.

1. Find a way to release it and move on:

   - I wrote a letter to him;
   - I confronted her (the other woman).

   A whole lot of things happened between those dashes that I didn't expect.

2. There is life after divorce. He was not happy. So, there really was no sense in me trying to hold on to someone who wasn't "happy".

   - I just wish it was done differently.
   - He was focused on getting me to "LET GO!!!...LET GO!!!...LET HIM GO!!!...

3. Have Periodic Moments of "Check-In" with your significant other: Is everything good?

   - Because things apparently change
   - And, people change

4. Ladies, you need to ... have a household account and a separate account – because he found a way to get money to move.

- I was thinkin' how do you have money to move – he sold a car my cousin had given us and I got very angry that we didn't split any of the money from the sale of that car. Hey, wasn't it **our** money from the sale of **my cousin's** car?

5. Let the Man be the Man. Enough said on that lesson.

6. You cannot love someone more than you love GOD or YOURSELF.

   - Was I placing my relationship with my husband over God?
   - Even if your weight isn't where you want it to be, you still have to love yourself first. YOU'VE GOTTA LOVE YOURSELF FIRST.
   - They were my world. My KIDS and my HUSBAND were the most IMPORTANT things in my life. Humm.... Did I LOVE them more than I LOVED GOD or even MYSELF?

CHAPTER 7
BREAST CANCER:
WHY ME? WHY NOT ME?

"You hear about it.
You know someone else who has it.
But you don't think it will happen to you."

The story of my being diagnosed with and then overcoming breast cancer could easily be told from the perspective of pain and suffering. Rather, since this is a book focused on encouraging women to have conversations about sensitive and critical topics that they normally would not have, I am taking the approach of an educator. Thus, my primary goal in this conversation on breast cancer is to educate and increase awareness. I want to reach as many individuals as possible across the country, and hopefully around the world, who are unaware of the signs, symptoms and preventative measures that can be taken with respect to breast cancer. In addition to educating and increasing awareness about breast cancer, I also want to inspire women who have been diagnosed with breast cancer to not give up: to not automatically take it as a death sentence.

The statistics related to women and breast cancer are alarming and overwhelming. They are highly indicative of an urgent need to increase public awareness. For example, there is an estimated "1 in 8 U.S. women (about 12.4%) who will develop invasive breast cancer over the course of her lifetime." {SOURCE: BreastCancer.org}

No. I will not bombard you with an endless list of statistics about breast cancer. I have reserved that for the Appendix section. What I believe is most important or the heart of this book is that I share with you what has proven to be my formula for success: how and why I believe I am a survivor of breast cancer. Simply stated, there are a number of essential ingredients that have made it possible for me to have survived breast cancer for 7 years and to be living a vibrant and fully active life.

Essential Ingredient #1: A strong relationship and belief in God. A belief that God will never leave you. A belief that God never fails. A belief that God has a purpose for our life.

Essential Ingredient #2: A long list of family and friends who were right by my side every step of the way.

Essential Ingredient #3: Maintaining a mindset that was focused more on living than on dying.

Essential Ingredient #4: Choosing to see myself as "powerful" rather than "powerless."

Cancer is one of those traumatic life events that any person can experience. It inevitably will force you to be honest with yourself about your belief in God or a Higher Power. Is God just this fictional character that lives far off in the clouds? Or, is God an active, living presence that embodies every part of your soul and being? I believe the latter—that God embodies every part of my soul and being.

My faith in God was greatly tested. Breast cancer stared me in the face, day after day, and dared me to prove that I believed in God. This is why it's so important for me to share with you the story of my being diagnosed with breast cancer, having a mastectomy, going through chemotherapy, radiation and being cancer-free for nearly seven years. By sharing my story, my hope is that it will plant in your mind and in your spirit seeds of hope, inspiration and practical guidance; and that, these seeds over time will take root, become fertile, and begin to blossom.

Why Me?

October 2013, at the age of fifty-five, I was still picking up the pieces from my divorce after 30 years of marriage. While my feelings of hurt, anger and betrayal were no longer lingering on the surface, I still was in a process of healing emotionally and psychologically. One of the things that preoccupied much of my time and energy was running my full-service marketing research business. The rest of my time was spent with family and friends.

It was during this time that I started becoming actively involved with the Center for Black Women's Wellness (CBWW) — a premier community-based family service center committed to improving the health and wellness of underserved black women and their families. In conjunction with my involvement with CBWW, I became familiar with Susan G. Komen Atlanta. Their mission is to promote greater awareness of breast cancer primarily by increasing the number of screenings which subsequently leads to earlier detection. For women diagnosed with breast cancer, Susan G. Komen Atlanta also supports research and facilitates access to quality care with the goal of increasing rates of survival. This includes providing resources and direct financial support by funding mammogram screenings for grassroot organizations such as the Center for Black Women's Wellness (CBWW).

I was first introduced to the CBWW several years prior while attending one of their Health Fairs. A friend, whose daughter was singing at the event, had invited me. Having signed up on their mailing list while attending the health fair, I periodically began to receive emails from them. In most instances, I never paid much attention to them. For some reason, when I received one of their emails in the spring of 2013, something about the flyer for the event caught my attention. It was announcing an upcoming Monthly Walk, and I instantly decided to attend.

These walks were generally held the third Saturday of the month at the foot of Stone Mountain Park. Every month the group walked around or hiked up Stone Mountain Park. So, it was not just a social gathering of men and women. It was encouraging everyone who attended to take care of their bodies and their overall health. As a result, I quickly became a regular.

During one particular walk, probably around September of 2013, I said out loud to myself, "You know.... It's time for me to get my mammogram." Having verbalized my thought out loud, the person walking alongside me overheard what I said. At the time, I had no idea that she was the person who was in charge of coordinating the scheduling of all mammograms for CBWW. The young woman hearing these words come out my mouth, turned to me and said, "Why don't you just come to the Center for Black Women's Wellness and get a mammogram?"

My immediate response was, "I don't have any medical insurance. I'm recently divorced and no longer have coverage since I was always on my husband's insurance."

She quickly informed me that the center has no restrictions on who can receive services; they help women who are underinsured or who have no insurance at all. If you have a job, the cost is only $25. If you're not working or don't have the means, it's free.

So very excited to hear this, one or two weeks later, on October 1st of 2013, I went to the Center for Black Women's Wellness. They were having a mobile mammography unit from St. Joseph Hospital set up right in their parking lot. After completing all the prerequisite paperwork, I then met with a Case Manager to complete the intake. Just as she promised, I only paid $25.

I remember them calling me back to the physician's room. To my surprise, I was seen by a Caucasian female physician. What a shock! I don't know why I only expected to see black physicians volunteering their time for a black organization.

In the beginning, the doctor asked me standard health questions as part of conducting a health assessment —you know weight, height, blood pressure, etc. They, then, gradually dug deeper into my medical history.

Next was the examination of my breasts. Having had a breast exam conducted before, I was totally comfortable with the procedure. Following the breast exam, the physician directed me outside to the St. Joseph's mobile unit for the actual mammogram. The entire process from intake to the mammogram was completed in about two hours.

Probably a week passed before I received the results by phone, which I thought was unusual. Typically, they just mail or email you something that basically says the results are "negative." However, when I received the call, they said they saw something on my X-Rays and wanted to take a closer look; they would like for me to come back in. However, this time they wanted me to go to the St. Joseph Breast Imaging Center.

Accompanied by my mom, they conducted the same breast exam and mammogram but took a lot more images and pictures. A couple days later I got another call. They said they saw something on my right breast but weren't sure what it was. So, they needed to do a biopsy (that is, take a sample from my right breast).

The biopsy procedure, unlike the basic mammogram, was very uncomfortable. You stick your right breast down into a cup-shaped container. Then, once it is perfectly placed, they have to numb it a little bit. This is because part of the biopsy procedure involves aspirating a portion of the breast tissue that can be taken to the lab for closer examination.

You have to lie flat on your stomach on a table and watch them insert a needle into your breast. When I heard a sudden pop and felt a jolt of pain, I thought I was going to jump up off the table. The pain was excruciating.

I quickly settled down only to realize that wasn't the end of it. They kept repeating the turning motion. And every time, I kept hearing a pop sound following continuous surges of pain. My speculation was that, despite numbing me before starting the invasive procedure, they were hitting a nerve which was causing the excruciating pain.

When they finished the procedure, they put a band-aid over the area. This was for any residual bleeding. I later discovered it was to cover a scar that was left from the procedure.

On a side note, in going through this procedure, I also learned a bit of history about Women's Rights. One of the female staff members informed me that years ago women had to fight in Congress for a law to be passed permitting the numbing of a woman's breast. Then, later in the week while attending my breast cancer support group, the topic came up again. When I shared my experience of going to the doctor for further examination and how uncomfortable and painful the procedure was, one of the group members kept saying how fortunate I am. She said, "Years ago, just think about what you just had done where they numbed you...Think about the number of women who had this procedure done without the numbing agent."

This sounded so ridiculous! Obviously, numbing of the breast is needed prior to administering because this is a very painful and invasive procedure. My reaction was one of total shock and disbelief. I said, "Girl, what!!! They had to fight to get that procedure done a different way? Oh My Goodness!!

Another week passed before I was called back to the doctor's office to hear the lab results from the biopsy. Anxious to hear what they would say, I disappointingly was told they would have to do further testing. This included having another mammogram. They told me they just weren't sure what was going on and subsequently needed to conduct more tests. By looking in their eyes, I could confirm that they truly were as perplexed as I was.

Believe it or not, at this point, I still wasn't feeling too concerned about what the outcome might be. The thought of having breast cancer had not entered my mind. I was just going about my daily routine of trying to keep up with my always hectic work and professional life.

I took my mom with me again for the next mammogram. When they called us into a room that appeared to look like a consultation room and not an exam room, we immediately could see a number of x-ray images hanging up. Suddenly, my heart started racing. I was like, "Oh, my God! This is not going to be good."

That was the first time I started to get nervous. Initially, however, I just thought they were being extra careful to make sure they didn't overlook anything. But now, I was beginning to fear the worst.

When the doctor entered the room and turned to talk to my mom and I, that's when everything went into slow motion. It was as though I went into a time warp. I will never forget the doctor's words. She said, "I have bad news and good news. You have breast cancer. It's stage zero."

That's when the big punch to the gut finally came. My heart sank, and there was a big lump in my throat.

As I slowly closed my eyes, attempting to fully absorb the life-changing news, my heart and spirit went to a very dark place reminiscent of when my ex-husband sat me down and told me he wanted a divorce. It was the weirdest feeling, to say the least, hearing the doctor deliver such news that was devastating yet positive all at once.

The devastating news was that I had breast cancer. The good news was that it was Stage Zero. This was something I had never heard of before. When I told the doctor I didn't know what they meant by Stage Zero, she explained that it's a term indicating that my cancer is at the lowest risk level possible. Higher risk levels are Stage 1, 2, 3 all the way up to Stage 4.

Taking in the good news is what made my heart and mood start to lighten up somewhat considering the circumstances. The Dr. continued by stating that certain procedures or medical treatments can be utilized depending upon the stage of the cancer. With my Stage Zero level, we, for example, had a number of treatment options including having a lumpectomy, and very likely without the need for chemotherapy or radiation treatment.

So, hearing the upside of my diagnosis, I left the doctor's office feeling fairly optimistic. At the same time, going to all these appointments and now knowing I would have to have major surgery, there was an increasing amount of stress about all the medical costs. I had already been getting bills in the mail. Now, with this diagnosis, it just meant several more, much larger medical bills were on the way.

Fortunately, once again, the Center for Black Women's Wellness came to the rescue and relieved me of all my medical expenses. From donated funds that are earmarked specifically to help individuals like myself who don't have insurance, they covered all of my bills. All I had to do was show them my receipts.

Their financial assistance was a tremendous relief. However, once I kept getting bills in the mail for $300, $500 and increasingly larger and larger amounts, I wasn't sure what to do. They were really starting to add up and with that came a greater sense of anxiety. But, the Center for Black Women's Wellness not only continued to step in providing direct financial assistance. They also made me aware of financial support provided by the State of Georgia that very few individuals ever hear of. This very special "free" healthcare assistance program is called "Emergency Women's Medicaid." It is only available to women who have no insurance and have been diagnosed with breast cancer, ovarian cancer, or cervical cancer.

Much of why many individuals (women) are unaware of this special state program is because it is only administered by the local Health Centers. That is, you have to go directly through a local health center in order to apply. The Center for Black Women's Wellness (CBWW) referred me to a local health center near a hospital, which at the time was called Georgia Baptist, now called Atlanta Medical Center (operated by WellStar Health Systems). All in one day, I filled out the paperwork, was evaluated by a case manager, and just like that was approved.

So, while there was a tremendous sense of relief in knowing that I didn't have to worry or stress financially about obtaining full medical treatment, I still had to contend with the psychological aspects of coming to grips with being diagnosed with breast cancer. I didn't go as far as thinking that I was cursed to get such a disease. I remained fairly optimistic by consciously doing everything I could to ensure that I didn't allow myself to become depressed.

It was like I was being bombarded with additional information about breast cancer from all directions. I actually received the final news of my actual diagnosis of breast cancer during the month of October which is Breast Cancer Awareness Month. Then, when calling my sister to break the news to her, I was informed that there is a history of breast cancer in our family; that we had three third cousins who died from it. While I had no idea what stage of breast cancer they had, the thought alone of it hitting so close to home added to my feelings of fear and anxiety about my own personal fate.

In an attempt to eliminate my fears and to educate myself in general about the disease, I reached out to some of my cousins, but they weren't able to give me any answers about how their relatives passed. What was even more disheartening was their avoidance of talking about the topic. It was like there was this big cloud or wall of secrecy where everyone was hush-hush about it; no one wanted to talk, and it really frustrated me. I was fighting a life-threatening disease and needed as much family history as possible.

Through my crash course introduction to breast cancer, I had quickly learned the significance of early detection (and family history)—that this literally could be the difference between life and death. So, to experience such avoidance of the topic among family members was very saddening.

Becoming more frustrated with the dead ends I was running into in trying to gather information from family members, I suddenly remembered a great resource that I had not yet thought to call upon. Having served on the Community Advisory Board of DeKalb Medical Center at Hillandale (now Emory – Hillandale), I had become acquainted with a renowned breast surgeon named Dr. Rosebud. Upon reaching out to her, Dr. Rosebud agreed to see me. But, she worked for DeKalb Medical Center, and my Emergency Women's Medicaid didn't cover medical costs at that facility. God, once again, however, was intervening and performing miracles on my behalf. Just when I thought I was faced with another insurmountable roadblock; it was quickly moved out of the way.

In talking through my payment options with Dr. Rosebud, she happened to mention that she also was on staff with Emory Hospital. And, I had quickly recalled that they were one of the Emergency Women's Medicaid approved medical facilities. So, now knowing that I had medical insurance to cover the examination and any future procedures, we went ahead and scheduled an appointment.

At my initial appointment with Dr. Rosebud, she said, "Listen. I need to know what I'm working with. The first thing we need to do is for me to see all of your medical records." So, I made it a priority to contact The Center for Black Women's Wellness and St. Joseph's Medical Center to obtain all my medical records.

After reviewing my medical records, Dr. Rosebud, then said, "Now that I know what I'm working with, I need you to get an MRI." She, then, requested another mammogram, which was taken in her office. Before I knew it, we were in Mid-November 2013.

When I was called in for my next appointment, my assumption was that it would just be to review the imaging and to schedule the lumpectomy to remove the lump in my breast. Never anticipating hearing any news worse than what I had already heard, I went alone to my next appointment.

Dr. Rosebud is in such high demand that it really is an adventure every time you go to her office. You have no idea if you'll be there for two hours or eight hours. You might arrive at 7:45am for an 8am appointment but not be seen until 2pm or 3pm in the afternoon. It's that unpredictable. What many people do is bring their laptops or tablets to work on or books to read. Otherwise, you could go crazy trying to kill time. The one major timesaver is that, rather than having to be referred out, her office is set up to conduct mammograms and most other small procedures.

For this appointment, I probably waited four hours to be seen. When I was finally called from the waiting room into an exam room, I sat there for probably twenty minutes. Dr. Rosebud walked in with her normal confident stride and serious tone. She first looked at the images hanging on the board before turning to me and saying, "Let me tell you what we're working with here." Both of our eyes turned to the hanging images where you could see the outlining of my breasts.

She then said, "I don't think you need a lumpectomy. You need a mastectomy."

I, without hesitation, blurted out, "That is not what I came in here for! I thought I was coming to see you to schedule my lumpectomy!"

She then said, "Do you see all these little white spots right here on your right breast?"

I said, "Yes."

She, then, pointed to them and said, "Those are calcification.... Now, not to throw out the possibility of them being cancerous, but they definitely can turn into it. I want to remove that risk."

She, then, continued, "There's so many of them that we can't remove all those calcifications. If we removed all of them, you know, it would be like removing your breast. So, I suggest you do a skin-sparing mastectomy."

With my jaw dropped to the floor, and mouth wide open, I just stared at her for a minute before finally saying, "Dr. Rosebud, in November I'm going to Jamaica! I go every year. And, I also have a friend who is taking me on a cruise from Christmas to New Year's." I had just started dating my current husband.

The Dr. looked at me, kind of processing what I had just told her, and said, "Well, you're stage zero.... That is a long way from stage 4 breast cancer. So, go ahead, do what you must do, and then, in January 2014, we'll do the mastectomy."

I looked at her once again, still in shock, but this time more receptive and accepting of the reality and necessity of what she was saying. "Ok Dr. Rosebud. If this is what you feel we need to do, then okay."

In my final words to the doctor, before leaving the office, I tried to project confidence. But as I headed back out through the waiting room towards the elevator, I was overcome with a feeling of nauseousness in my gut. My head was spinning, and I really needed to sit down to take a moment to compose myself. But my emotions and adrenaline were running so high that I just kept walking at a fast pace.

Just as I was about to exit out of the doctor's office, two familiar faces bumped right into me as they were entering this same doctor's office. It was a church member of more than twenty years. She was escorting her elderly mother to the doctor's office for an appointment. Once we made direct eye contact, their entire body language shifted from calm and relaxed to tense and concerned. Before saying anything, they gave me that look like, "What's wrong?"

I answered their question without them even having to ask me a second time. I just blurted out "I need a mastectomy!!! That's not what I came here for. But I need a mastectomy!!!"

You could feel a sense of instant grief overcome them. In an attempt to comfort me, they replied, "Oh, we're so sorry! We'll be praying for you."

I don't recall the walk from exiting the doctor's office to actually sitting in my car. I don't even remember saying goodbye to the members from my church. I only recall feeling too paralyzed by the emotion of fear to start my car and to drive out of the parking lot. I was too emotionally fragile to get behind the wheel. So, I just sat there with my head down crying.

My mind was on autopilot. It just kept playing the doctor's words over and over: "I don't think you need a lumpectomy. You need a mastectomy... I don't think you need a lumpectomy. You need a mastectomy."

How could this be happening to me? That's all I kept thinking to myself. We read and hear about celebrities and people we know dying of cancer. We see the commercials promoting fundraising events to conduct research on finding a cure and to increase awareness, but you never think it's going to happen to you. Or should I say, I never thought it would happen to ME.

With each passing moment, my feelings of self-pity were expanding further and further. The reality of losing one of my breasts was starting to sink in. I was already beginning to feel that I was less of a woman. My breasts are one of the most sensual arousing parts of my body that I love to be stimulated; the heightened arousal of a sexual experience would never be the same.

The first person I called after leaving the doctor's office was my mother. "Everything is going to be alright" were the first words out of her mouth. I, then, called my sister. Her words were equally comforting.

Then, without consciously deciding to drive there, I found myself sitting in the parking lot of Walmart near Stonecrest Mall. The next person I picked up the phone and called was Pete. We had only been dating for 6 months, but to call him at such a dire moment was a clear indication of how strong of a bond we had formed in such a short amount of time.

When Pete answered the phone, he instantly knew that something wasn't right. So, he asked, "What's wrong?

I replied, "I just came from the doctor, and I have to get a mastectomy! I'm getting ready to lose my right breast."

Before he could attempt to comfort me, I yelled out, "You didn't ask for this!!!"

Not hesitating for even a second, he immediately replied, "Baby, I'm in it for the long haul."

A flood of tears began to rush from my eyes as my head sunk into my hands.

I don't remember how long we stayed on the phone. I just know it was a pivotal moment in our relationship, one in which I knew that we were no longer just boyfriend and girlfriend; that he was going to be my future husband. Not just because God had placed him in my life to be an anchor. Because time and time again, Pete proved to be a man of his word, a highly honorable man.

We, for example, just as scheduled, still went on our cruise. It didn't matter to him if I had a death sentence. He loved me for me and, through his actions, was showing that he truly was in it for the long haul. I just had to let go of the past, trust him, and allow him to be the man he desired to be in my life.

We had such a good time on our cruise that I can easily say it was one of the best trips of my life. More importantly, going on the cruise and taking my annual Mission Trip to Jamaica in December set the stage for me to continue maintaining a sense of normalcy in my life despite the diagnosis. More than anything, family, friends and Pete being there day and night to support and encourage me helped me keep my sanity.

Not long after I received my diagnosis, I asked my sister when was the last time that she had gotten her mammogram. After much thought, she said, "1 think I've had one but 1 can't remember the last time." That's when, I said, "Girl, you better go to the doctor and get a mammogram!" Low and behold she hadn't been in five years.

They immediately saw something on her mammogram, had her wait to talk to another doctor to review her x-rays, and she cried the whole time explaining why she was there. She said it was because her sister who had just been diagnosed with breast cancer had encouraged her to get her mammogram.

Wow! Fortunately, she listened and scheduled an appointment right away. A few weeks later my sister called and asked if I was sitting down. That's when she broke the news to me that she was diagnosed with stage two breast cancer. The ending to this story could have been much worse had there not been early detection. Instead of losing her life, she only had to get a lumpectomy.

The lives of my sister and I intersected in a strange way. We were both going through chemo and radiation at the same time. I was in Atlanta, and she was in Akron, Ohio. While heartbreaking, the upside was that we were able to support one another. And, more of our family members and close friends were getting screened.

FaceTime technology was a lifesaver. It allowed my sister and I to connect through videoconferencing while going through months of treatment and recovery; this was especially significant during some of the roughest times when our hair was falling out and we were going bald. Often, we didn't even talk about breast cancer. Some days, we would just tell jokes and laugh. This was therapeutic in and of itself.

The two months leading up to my scheduled surgery quickly passed. I had mentally prepared myself for it only to have it delayed on two different occasions, both times due to weather (ice storms). So, instead of having my surgery January 2014, I checked into Emory University Hospital Midtown for my surgery in February of 2014.

I was told that, even though the surgery required an overnight stay, it was fairly straightforward. In performing the surgery, it required two surgeons. Dr. Rosebud performed the skin-sparing mastectomy and removed my right breast and then Dr. Daisy, my plastic surgeon followed her and inserted an expander that was shaped much like a plastic water bottle. As promised, I was in and out in less than 36 hours.

Following the surgery with Dr. Rosebud, she then provided me with aftercare instructions and a referral appointment with the plastic surgeon. This was because I had elected to have reconstructive surgery. The plastic surgeon was Dr. Daisy. She came highly recommended by Dr. Rosebud. The expander was inserted so that, once fully awake, my chest would not be totally flat.

I left the hospital with two drainage tubes that needed to be emptied, and the amount of fluid needed to be measured daily. I was also told I would have the results back from the procedure in a few days. So, I waited. A few day later, the news I received from Dr. Rosebud was not good. She discovered some concerns with the test results.

I was diagnosed with Triple Negative Breast Cancer, which means I tested negative to estrogen, negative to progesterone and negative to HER-2. This indicated that I no longer was stage zero, I now was diagnosed with triple negative breast cancer stage 2. It makes me think that the cancer must have been in my body longer than I realized because there had been no visible signs or symptoms; I had no lumps, bumps, or drainage. Without early detection from a routine mammogram, there's no telling how the cancer might have advanced in my body before being discovered. **That's why it is so important to have yearly mammograms.**

What made the current news even more perplexing was that when Dr. Rosebud removed the right breast, she also removed most of the lymph nodes on the right side as well. There was cancer in one of the lymph nodes—not in all but still there. So, there was total confidence that any traces of cancer were completely removed during the surgery.

Given traces of cancer were still present, even after removing one of my breasts, the new priority now was to see an oncologist. And, this meant I was going to have to have chemo. I was quite shaken up because having chemo meant I was going to lose my hair. For me, at that time, my hair was not just an expression of my femininity; it was a fashion statement. I had beautiful locks that I would wrap on top of head.

When meeting with the oncologist, I was still trying to hold on to a glimmer of hope that I would not lose my hair. My spirit was energized in discovering that Dr. Moss, my oncologist, was a wonderful African-American woman. Within minutes of meeting her, I anxiously asked, "What are the chances my hair will fall out?" and she said, "100%."

All I could see in my mind was images of my locks falling out while I was in the shower, followed by me screaming in horror and breaking down crying. However, I quickly embraced the inevitable and just went ahead and cut my hair to a low cut. I chose to keep my locks by storing them in a bag because I just didn't want to lose that part of me.

I started chemotherapy in May of 2014, and yes, my hair did fall out. However, it was very important to me to go to my chemo appointments looking good. So, I would put on makeup and get dressed up just to help myself feel better, to still feel beautiful as a woman.

Chemotherapy was grueling, frequently filled with extremely long days. You first sign in, wait, get your blood drawn, and have your vitals like blood pressure checked to make sure that they are within a certain range. You also have to wait on the results from the blood draw to ensure all your numbers are in an acceptable range. Otherwise, you would not be able to receive treatment that day. Then, of course, this is followed by more and more waiting.

They, then, take you back to the therapy room and give you IV's full of antibiotics and nausea medication, even before administering the chemo medicine. More waiting before you go home to make sure you are feeling well.

The next day I had to go back to get a Neulasta injection in my stomach. Now, you no longer have to go back the next day. They invented a Neulasta patch which releases the medicine at the proper time.

The first set of chemo treatments were fine. It was the second regime of drugs that, once they hit my blood steam, immediately caused me to have neuropathy in my feet. It's a long-term side effect I still live with today. So, it was not just mentally and physically draining. It was taking a physical toll on my body. Nevertheless, my mindset was: if this is the one side-effect I have to live with, so be it. Thank You God for Deliverance and Healing!

I also need to mention that chemo and radiation can take a toll on your heart. Every 3 months, I see a magnificent cardiologist, Dr. Petals. This is to keep a check on that valuable part of our body, the heart. Again, if this is one of the side-effects I have to live with, so be it. Thank You God for Deliverance and Healing!

One more organization that I must mention in my book is Turning Point Breast Cancer Rehabilitation located in Roswell, Georgia. Turning Point Breast Cancer Rehabilitation is a non-profit 501(c)3 organization that improves the quality of life for women with breast cancer by providing, promoting and advocating specialized and evidence-based rehabilitation. If you recall, Dr. Rosebud removed most of the lymph nodes under my right arm after having my right breast removed. As a result, there was limited mobility in that right arm.

Well, Turning Point was amazing at helping me to use that right arm again. They have physical therapists to guide you through your healing journey. You can get massages as well as nutritional tips. They also provided me with compression garments at a reduced cost (sleeves) for both my right hand and arm. I use them on long flights to help with swelling (avoiding lymphedema). They also measured my right arm just in case it starts to swell in the future (Lymphedema refers to swelling and is most commonly caused by the removal of or damage to your lymph nodes as part of cancer treatment.) Lymphedema can come at any time and there is no cure at this time.

I finished chemo in August 2014. I remember wanting to go on my annual Mission Jamaica trip in December and asking the Radiologist if this was possible. He said we would be cutting it close, but he expedited my appointments to get fitted for my breast covering (when you have radiation, they custom fit an apparatus that you put over you for protection during the radiation procedures).

Just in time, I finished my radiation treatments the Tuesday before Thanksgiving, November 2014. Due to the total number of radiation treatments (30, I went everyday, 5 days a week for 6 weeks), I got third degree burns on my neck and underarms. Also, sometimes the blood circulation periodically just slows down, and my feet cramp up. I also endured numerous reconstructive surgeries. Again, I must say, if this is one of the side-effects I must live with, so be it. Thank You God for deliverance and healing!

Without questions, I had to overcome a lot. In the end, I not only survived. I am living a full life. So, for that, I Thank and Praise God!!!

At some point, I started participating in a breast cancer support group. There were several men and women who were suffering far worse than I was. I mean literally every day for them was life and death. I still was very mobile and able to work and engage in daily activities. Many of the other group members could barely walk or were always in a constant state of pain. Seeing this provided me with a great source of inspiration. They not only were courageous. They shared a lot of wisdom, deep insights and made profound statements such as: "I had breast cancer, but breast cancer didn't have me."

Within months of ending chemotherapy, I also saw how my trials and tribulations proved to be an inspiration for other women to be proactive in getting screened (in getting their mammogram). My baby sister, for one, said I saved her life. She went on to say that, if I had not been diagnosed, she would not have gotten her mammogram. But, from my perspective, it wasn't me. It was God, because God never fails.

Not until recently, in the process of writing this book, was I reminded of a number of other women who were encouraged or inspired by me to schedule a mammogram. One of the most touching stories is the niece of one of my close friends. Her life was saved because of early detection. After getting a mammogram, it was discovered that her cancer was so advanced they would have to remove both of her breasts. In the words of her aunt:

> *Your conversation with my niece played a huge*
> *role in her making the decision to have her double*

mastectomy. She's in remission and I can never thank you enough for having that difficult conversation with her so she could make an informed decision.

Overall, experiencing being diagnosed with, treating and fighting to overcome breast cancer was a nightmare! Yet, I hate to imagine how emotionally painful the process would have been for me had I not had an amazing support system. For many individuals fighting cancer, they have no one or maybe only one person who unwaveringly are right by their side through all of the treatments and sad and depressed days of feeling self-doubt and self-pity. I was extremely fortunate to have more individuals than I can count on both hands showering me with love, food, flowers, cards, money, visits and steadfast support through this ordeal. So, whenever I have the opportunity to give words of encouragement or advice to someone going through what I've gone through, I do it.

In the end, God gave me the victory. Because I kept the faith, never ceased to pray, and walked with my head held high, God Delivered ME. Thanks to my husband Pete, my mom Gloria and a host of family and friends for standing right by my side! Thank You Lord for Delivering ME!

Lessons Learned from Fighting Breast Cancer

1. Maintain a sense of normalcy in your life despite the diagnosis.

2. Early Detection is the key. Get screened at the age of 40 or sooner if you have a history of Breast Cancer.

3. Family History is important. When possible, try to find out if there is a history of Cancer in your family. I know we don't always like to talk about what causes deaths in our family, but it really is important to know.

4. Follow your doctor(s) regimen. You will have several types of doctors. Make all your appointments (try not to miss any doctor appointments).

5. Let your physician(s) know when you are NOT feeling well. If you are hurting or don't feel well, don't be AFRIAD to ASK QUESTIONS.

6. Keep a positive attitude. There will be times when you are so sick you can't lift your head off the pillow and you don't want to eat, but still .... Try and Keep a POSITIVE ATTITUDE.

7. Once again, the three most important things I want to leave you with, that I know to be true are:

   - God will never leave you.
   - God never fails.
   - God has a purpose for our life.

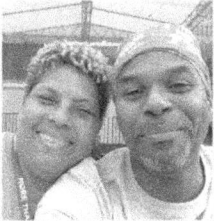 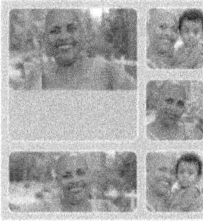 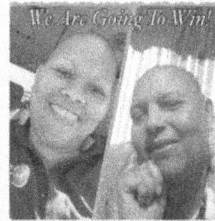

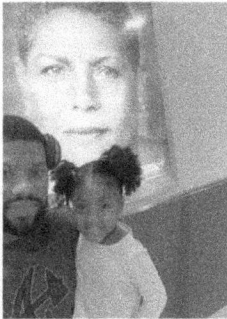 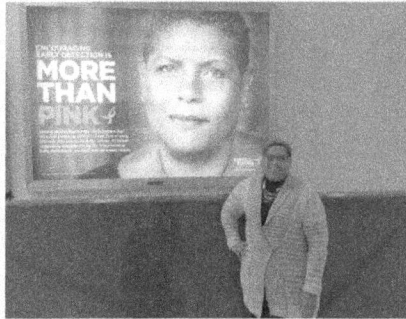

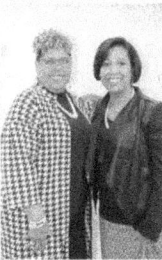 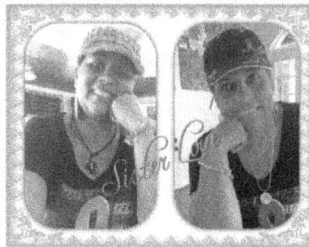

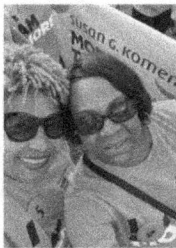 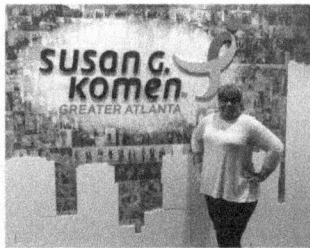

Woman 2 Woman

CHAPTER 8
FINDING NEW LOVE

Love is a powerful life force. Few find true love once in their lifetime. I am fortunate to have found love twice.

For many individuals, if the relationship ends due to infidelity or simply from growing apart, it's hard for them to believe that true love ever existed. But, that's how I've learned to look at it; that my first husband really did love me, that he truly was in love with me for a number of years. There just was a turning point in our relationship where it got away from us and we were never able to get it back on track.

Going through my divorce, while gut wrenching, in the long-term proved to be life-changing for the better. It forced me to open and discover an entirely new sense of liberation. For one, the self-conscious feelings about my weight that I had harbored for years were becoming less of a burden. Secondly, having slept with only one man my entire life, I found the courage to give myself permission to explore who I was sexually. While I'm not going to say I was promiscuous, I would say that, over a period of a few years, I allowed myself to go against my religious beliefs since childhood.

The reality was that, once I had given myself ample time to grieve the ending of my marriage, I adopted the attitude that this was my time to finally be free and to have fun. I viewed it as the beginning of a new season of my life. So, to say the least, getting married again was the last thing on my mind. Most importantly, having been such a giver for most of my life—sacrificing so much of myself for my children and my husband—I wanted a man in my life who could be just as attentive to my needs as I was to his.

The point I'm trying to make is that I wasn't looking for Mr. Right. What was most important to me at that time of my life (in 2011, 2012) was having fun and being pampered, or at least dating a man who I could feel was really into me. In my first marriage, I was the giver. So, even just for the purposes of dating, I was adamant about being with someone who was eager to focus their attention on making me "happy", doing for me.

In May of 2013, however, there was another monumental shift in my life. While I still wasn't focused on finding Mr. Right, he just suddenly appeared out of nowhere. Well, actually, he was introduced to me by his Divorce Attorney, which happened to be an old friend of mine. All she said to me was that there was this guy who was going through a divorce and she was representing him. She, then, asked if she could give him my number. He sounded like a nice guy, and I trusted my friend's judgment. So, I said, "Sure."

He called me within 24 hours. One of the first things that impressed me about him was that, during our very first conversation, he said he preferred to finalize the filing of his divorce papers with the court before we talked further. He expressed that he would love to get to know me better but had to deal with his divorce first. Knowing that I was still on vacation with some girlfriends and then headed to Akron for my niece's graduation, I said "Okay."

A couple weeks later, when I returned from the graduation, I received a call from him. We immediately connected and talked for hours. Shortly thereafter, we went on our first date, which probably was the first weekend in June. It was on a Saturday. The same day as our first date I had a sorority event. I remember telling some of my sorority sisters that we needed to wrap up our meeting early because I had a blind date.

We met at Outback Steakhouse in Conyers, Georgia. I arrived a few minutes before him and sat in my car anxiously wondering what he would look like. Upon greeting each other, I was pleasantly surprised with his physical appearance. This made me feel even more at ease knowing that there was physical chemistry. As a result, the rest of the evening flowed naturally.

Dinner went so well that I accepted his invitation to continue the date by going to Bruster's for ice cream. Before I knew it, another hour had gone by. We effortlessly talked about a variety of topics including how our attorney friend had hooked us up on this date. He also showed his humorous side when sharing that Pete is his nickname and not actually his legal name.

Then, the heaviest subject of the evening finally came up. There is a ten-year age difference between the two of us. When we met, Pete was 45 and I was 55. While I expressed major concern about my being much older than he is, Pete quickly brushed it off like it was no big deal. Despite continuing to feel somewhat skeptical that this might become a bigger issue down the road, Pete's quiet sense of confidence and how comfortable I felt with him convinced me to let go and take him at his word.

That Saturday night, we ended our date on such a high that he surprised me by coming to my church the very next morning. This particular Sunday I was leading Praise and Worship. Imagine the look on my face when I scanned the audience and saw him sitting on the back row. Actually, it brought a smile to my face and I thought: Who does that after the first date? I thought it was so sweet.

Following church, we then went to the movies followed by dinner. At dinner, it became even more evident to me how great of a listener Pete was because the night before he had heard me say how much I really wanted to go see a new movie that had just been released. And, he took the initiative to bring up going to see this particular movie.

In a short period of time, probably within a couple of weeks, Pete was bold enough to ask me if we could officially start seeing each other. Despite our significant age difference, he was open to seeing where things could progress between us. He didn't necessarily ask to be boyfriend-girlfriend, but he made it clear that he's not the type of guy to date a lot of women. I loved hearing him clarify why he wanted to be direct and upfront regarding his intentions.

I didn't perceive his gesture as moving too fast. I viewed it as a sign of tremendous maturity and said, "Yes. I would love for us to see each other on a regular basis." It just so happened that we crossed paths at the right time, and I was finally ready to consider entering into another serious relationship.

The way things turned out I never dated another guy again, and Pete and I have been together ever since June 2013. The timing was good on his end as well because his divorce was final just two months later in August 2013. We hit such a stride in our relationship that he asked me to go to the courthouse with him on the date of his final divorce hearing. His wife did not appear in court, and as expected, the judge approved everything. His divorce was final and he was a free man.

Just as my friends and family had been there for me so many times through my divorce, I wanted to do something special for Pete. I know the emotional toll that going through a divorce can have on you. So, I wanted to help him take his mind off everything.

Yvetta, a close friend whom I call my God-Sister, helped me surprise Pete with a one-night getaway. We got him there by saying she had a client who was a famous entertainer needed her to stop by their hotel room to pick up something. She wanted us to meet her there so she could introduce us to this famous entertainer. Yvetta probably gave us the name of some famous person like Jill Scott, because that is Pete's all-time favorite female artist.

Anyway, when we opened the door, the room was lit up with candles and rose petals that led to the foot of the bed. Pete was totally taken by surprise and felt an even greater sense of disbelief in discovering that I had already packed his travel bag (to stay for the night). She even had a bottle of chilled wine and a basket of fruit and chocolates. Pete and I still remember that weekend as one of our most romantic and memorable weekends ever.

Also, in the month of August, I had planned a huge 80th Birthday Party for my father at a really nice seafood restaurant. Pete was my date. However, within minutes of picking me up, just as we were driving out of the subdivision, he received a call from his youngest daughter. I could hear her crying through the phone. That's when I told him to turn the car around to take me back to my house so that I could drive my car to the party. My parental instinct kicked in and I could tell it was one of those moments where he needed to be there for his daughter as a father. So, I just told him to go and be with his daughter; that it was alright not to attend the party.

Pete didn't make it to the party, but he called me that night and said he could not believe how well I handled the situation. More specifically, he couldn't believe that I didn't get an attitude, upset or jealous at all. That he appreciated I didn't give him an ultimatum. He went on to verbally express how amazing of a woman I was and that he was so glad to have me in his life. While I accepted his compliments, I told him that his daughter was in a time of need and that I understood he needed to be there as a parent.

Our relationship continued to grow stronger and stronger. That December we went on a Carnival cruise together and celebrated New Year's Eve. What is most significant about this is that Pete's spirit was one in which he would not let me get down on myself even though I had been diagnosed with cancer a few months earlier. Even more, my treatment would require that I undergo chemotherapy and have a mastectomy (that my right breast would have to be surgically removed). None of this, however, deterred him from continuing to pursue me and to convey his unwavering love and belief that we were meant to be together (meant to be husband and wife); even more importantly, that I would fully heal.

After we returned from the cruise, as scheduled, I had my surgery (mastectomy), in February 2014. I, then, started chemo in March 2014. My chemo treatments continued until August 2014 followed by radiation in October and November of that same year.

Through all of these treatments, Pete was right there. Because he never wavered, I was finally starting to believe that I not only might kick this disease, but that there would be a fairytale ending to our love story.

Getting Married

Neither of us were in a rush to get married again even though we both were open to it and desired it. Meeting someone new whom I could fall in love with again had always felt like a possibility. What I least expected was to live with a man I was not married to. Partly due to the fact that he spent so much time over my house, and also because it made economic sense, Pete moved in with me May 2015. Then, more than a year later, November 20, 2016, we got married.

Pete proposed to me on Christmas day 2015. It was supposed to be a surprise because he didn't want me to open my gift until later on that day during family dinner. However, because I was pouting he let me open my gift early. Although I spoiled his surprise, I will cherish that memory forever. We actually had two ceremonies. One of the ceremonies was on November 20, 2016 in a lovely home in Buckhead, Georgia. No, not the Buckhead you're thinking of north of downtown Atlanta. This Buckhead was in the beautiful countryside about an hour drive East of Atlanta towards Augusta. Having served on the board of Unconditional Love for Children (ULC), one of the board members is a minister. She graciously opened her home and hosted our wedding. She said, "All I need you to do is bring the dessert and I will do the rest.

It was supposed to be an intimate crowd, but as the date drew closer, it got bigger and bigger. Every time I called and gave her a number, she was so kind and said, "okay." It was going to be in her backyard near the lake, but on this particular day in November, it was very, very cold. So, we had to move the ceremony indoors.

OMG – when we walked into her house, she had transformed her den area into a chapel. I mean, she laid it out. The chairs were covered, candles for lighting and any and everything you could image at a typical wedding ceremony. She even gave each of us a room to change in. I, of course, got her master bedroom, and Yvetta did my make-up. The minister's sister served as the wedding coordinator, and all I can say is "What a Beautiful ceremony it was!" After the ceremony, we had a sit-down dinner also catered by the minister. Once again, she put everything together perfectly!

Two weeks later we were headed to Montego Bay, Jamaica on my annual Board Meeting and mission trip for Unconditional Love for Children (ULC). Well.... I always said that I wanted to get married by the beach and it happened. We actually wrote vows and the same beautiful minister who officiated our wedding ceremony in Buckhead was gracious enough to officiate this one as well. While she did say a special prayer over us, she also let us recite our own original vows (we had recited traditional vows at her home).

Usually, about 35 - 40 people attend the mission trip. Everyone who attended the mission trip that year was invited to the ceremony. It was held in a beautifully decorated Gazebo at the Half Moon Resort. Afterwards, we went back to the Villa's for a special dinner. It was absolutely an amazing week for us.

I still wanted to share our love as a couple with so many other people. Space was limited at the location of our ceremony in Buckhead, and many people don't attend or were unable to travel to Jamaica for a ceremony. So, the following year, June 2015, we had a big celebration of love at the Porter Sanford Performing

Arts Center in Decatur, Georgia. We had nearly 200 guests. That took some planning, but I had help from a wonderful party planner. When we walked in on that Red Carpet to Bruno Mars "24 Karat Magic," I almost started crying when I saw how beautifully she had decorated the atrium.

The reception included food, a wonderful dessert table and of course an open bar. There also was a DJ. So, everyone danced. A friend of mine sang us a song, and some of my sorority sisters from Delta Sigma Theta Sorority, Inc. even sang to me.

Pete often teases me and says we had three weddings. I always come back and say, "No – we had a traditional wedding. We then had a vow ceremony. And then, we had our reception."

Pete is an incredible man in more ways than I can count. He still opens doors, including car doors and he often cooks breakfast and serves it to me in bed. He not only laughs with me. He's able to cry with me.

Ultimately, I not only found true love in my husband Frederick Cornelius Taylor – "Pete", I found a life partner. I found someone who sees me as an equal and who truly understands me and accepts me for who I am.

Pete appearing in my life was a miracle from God. God knew what I needed and when I was going to need it. The reality, however, is that I would not have been ready to receive this blessing if I had not learned to forgive and to let go of all the hurt from the past. Scriptures from the Bible taught me forgiveness. Even more, there was a book I read by Colin Tipping called Radical Forgiveness. It totally opened my eyes to see and understand the power of forgiveness from a totally new perspective.

In Tipping's book, he talks about true forgiveness. He convincingly argues that forgiveness is the cornerstone for a loving heart and a peaceful life. Because, as long as you hold resentment and anger about things that happened in the past, they will continue to upset you in the present. Thus, you will never find peace.

Another major point of emphasis by the author is that when we have very painful breakups, our tendency is to automatically think that the long-term outcome will only be bad. However, Colin Tipping challenges you to stop and think that perhaps God did something "for you" instead of "something to you." Rather, through your pain, God may have given you something invaluable, that in the long run was for your good.

This entirely new philosophy on experiencing crisis in my life enabled me, for one, to let go of my pain and hurt from the past. Secondly, it helped me to realize that God had led, directed Frederick "Pete" Taylor into my life at precisely the right moment in time. That, once I was ready to receive this life altering blessing, God provided me with my true soul mate. God provided me with a man who would love me, cherish me and treat me as the QUEEN that I am!

Lesson on Finding New Love

1. Strive to find love within yourself first before you try to find it in someone else.

2. When you're blessed to find love again in your life, don't just look at the faults of the other person in earlier relationships. Fully examine yourself and what you could have done better. View the second time around with love as a gift not just for you to be loved and treated better, but for you to be a better partner and mate.

3. Being on the dating scene, you have to be careful. I did some dating through social media, but I eventually deleted my profile. I found that I am not a social media type of person. More than anything, I think it's best to approach it with the mindset of letting the man pursue you.

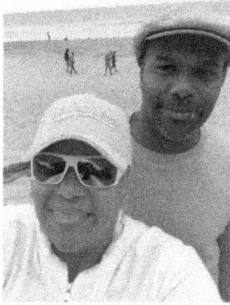
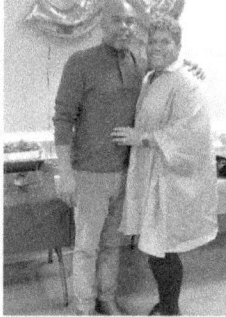
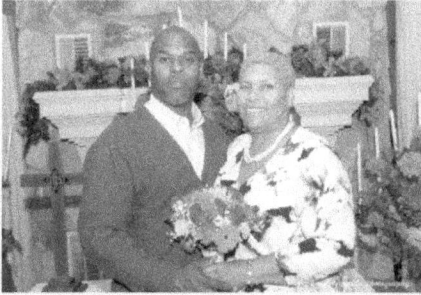
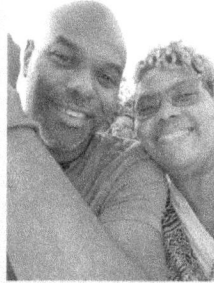
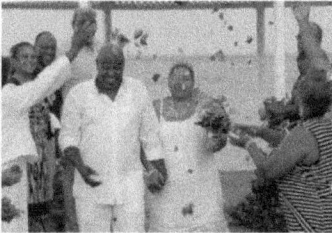
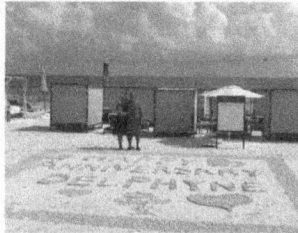
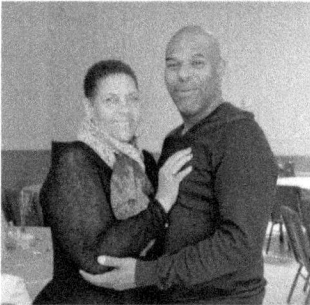
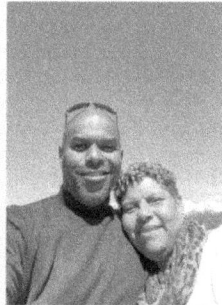

Woman 2 Woman

CHAPTER 9
FRIENDSHIP

What is Friendship?

Frequently in life, we don't realize how much someone means to us until they're no longer here. Maybe there is a major transition in our life, and we go to pick up the phone to call them when we suddenly remember they're no longer physically with us. Maybe we unconsciously get restless during a certain time of the year because it's nearing their birthday. Or, maybe, we just miss having a kindred spirit who enjoys talking about and doing the same things we enjoy.

When I thought about the *Woman 2 Woman* heartfelt conversations and circles that I hope this book will inspire, I felt that as we neared the end of this book, it would be important to touch on this subject. Talking about friendship was not a part of the original manuscript and outline of the book, but when I lost one of my closest friends right in the middle of writing the book, I knew then that something would be missing, or that the book would be incomplete, without discussing truly how valuable and significant it is to have quality people, and more specifically, quality friends in our lives. Yes, being in a circle with other women is good and greatly needed. However, there is something much more special about the personal one-on-one relationships we share with other women.

Secondly, I think that many of us have friends that really don't fall in the definition of what I would call friends. Rather, they are simply acquaintances. Why is it even important for me to point this out and challenge you to make a clear distinction? The answer is because friends play an important role in our life journey. Even more, when we decide that we want to be our best selves and fully commit to reaching our full potential, we can't have people in our inner circle who are just along for the ride. I'm not saying they have to be rich or geniuses or even beautiful. But they must have a clear sense of value. The kind of value in which it is undeniable that they are a blessing in our life and make the road that much easier rather than simply an additional weight we choose to carry all because we have so called "history."

On the flip side, when you look in the mirror and ask yourself, "Am I bringing value to the lives of the people I call friends, or who consider me their friend?" "Am I making the road easier and lighter for those who have granted me access and the privilege of being in their inner circle?

By no means do I wish to appear boastful or arrogant for being an exceptional person who lifts and inspires others. I simply am saying we should celebrate those who do live in such a way, because too frequently I see us as sisters tearing and dragging each other down.

As s a testimonial to the power of living our lives in this manner without seeking recognition or admonishment, I would like to share something that deeply moved me. It's excerpts from what my friend's daughter, Mekyah, said at her mother's homegoing service which inspired me to write this chapter on "Friendship." It epitomizes the thoughtful, kind, generous friend her mother Fern was. She consistently reciprocated what was given to her and never had a mindset of taking more than she gave.

My friend, Fern McQueen transitioned at the end of last year (2019). Her homegoing service was this past January 2020, and I spoke at her homecoming service. You will see excerpts from my words as well at the end of this chapter on "Friendship."

Anyway, here first are excerpts from part of what Mekyah shared at her mom's homecoming service:

I am warmly and happily accepting as my inheritance and my legacy, the ideal and practice of friendship. The ability to make friends, to nurture and maintain friendships across the span of multiple decades. Some for so long that your children forge a bond and then their children form bonds that are meaningful.

This practice of friendship is an important, securely understated and valuable idea that I have inherited from my mother. And I have decided that a part of my mother's legacy is what I now do with these bonds and my own.

To my mother's friends:

You are my inheritance. Whether your friendship traces back to growing up with mommy in Baxter Terrace, or if you were friends with mommy at Winston-Salem, if your mommy's friends from Spelman or you walked with her along the spiritual path that began at First African – my mother was intentional about nurturing her relationships.

She valued her friendships with you and in her I and my sister are the beneficiaries of that bond. When I think about my own friendships and the way they enrich my life, I am truly thankful to all of you for being that for my mom.

It is a testament to who mommy was as a friend and I will always have that to draw on as in my own friendships.

156

Mommy was intentional about reaching out, checking in, and making time.

Her legacy, in action, will be in the ways in which I am intentional about maintaining connections with her friends – not because it's what she would have wanted, but because it's what I want. In action, my mother's legacy is in the way I strengthen my own friendships and remain open to new connections and meaningful bonds. I am so thankful to you, mommy, for this incredible lesson on how to be – that I never ever knew I was learning. Love You Mom!

This is why I had to write a chapter on "Friendship" because Fern was such a true friend and an amazing overall person. As her daughter Mekyah said, she was intentional about her friendships, and I want to be that way as well.

As we close this chapter, I would like to share with you the words I spoke at Fern's homecoming service which was absolutely beautiful.

Fern McQueen:

Rest in Peace My Sister. I don't even remember how long I've known Fern and I don't remember when we established that I was her L'il Sis. I would call her Big Sis. I just know it's been a long time.

I could stand here and tell you so many stories about Fern, some really funny ones. Like one time on a cruise, every time we turned around Fern was asleep...When we were waiting at a doc to catch a ferry, she was sleep...When we were at the beach, Fern was sleep.

And, most recently, we went on a JUGS trip (that stands for "Just Us Girls Société": a traveling group started by another close friend of mine, Falisha Riaye). We take an annual trip every year. One time, we were playing a game of Taboo and Fern's word was "Hardwood Floors." Yet, every time she pronounced it, it sounded like "Harvard Floors." So, always being a comedian, the next year Fern brought all of us a piece of tile.

On a serious note, I'm friends with one of the news anchors in Atlanta and she asked me to speak during breast cancer month at her Church during "Worship in Pink" Sunday. I thought I was just going to say a few words and ended up delivering the morning sermon. Anyway, I told no one, not even my children that I would be speaking. I had only told my husband Pete and Fern and they made it into the introduction of my speech:

I am truly humbled right now. It is an honor and privilege to be here with you this morning.

I also want to recognize my wonderful, amazing Husband Pete (You'll hear more about him) and my Sistah/Friend – Fern, who walked with me through this Breast Cancer Journey.

Over the years, Fern became what I now call, "My Wisdom." We've had countless conversations on all types of subject matters. Many of you here have walked with me along my journey and I don't want to discount it, but Fern …. My Fern …. My Wisdom.

She would have those conversations with you and would not hold back or be afraid to tell you how she felt, or what she thought. But... at the same time would let you make the final decision. Sometimes I made the right decision and sometimes I didn't, but whatever happened, she would be right there with me, either rejoicing or encouraging me.

Fern is the reason that I am writing a book about my journey. When I was going through my journey with Breast Cancer, she gave me a journal with beautiful butterflies on the front of it. If anyone knows Fern, she loved butterflies. She gave me a card along with a journal that said:

Lil Sis,

I've been told that writing down the expressions we have during our life's journey helps us to really appreciate how far God has brought us when we look back and try to reflect.

I'm ever so sure that God is going to provide you with an awesome testimony that He wants you to share about Hope, Faith, His Goodness, Grace & Mercy.

I'm giving you this journal which ironically is called the "Tree of Life."

Please try to write about your journey. I don't want you to forget one minute of it as you share your testimony. You know that God answers the prayers of the righteous and you are surrounded by religious Prayer Warriors.

Love You Much,

Big Sis

She gave me this in 2014. I have several entries that started in March, but I must confess, my last entry is July of that same year. A lot has happened since then and she and I have had many, many conversations. I promise you Fern, I will pick up this Journal and begin writing again.

Fern knew that I began writing a book because of her. Well, what a joy and testimony to her spirit of love, encouragement and inspiration that the book is almost complete. We are in the final stages of editing.

Another person I would like to acknowledge in this chapter on friendship is Anthony Parnell. His family and friends from his hometown of Akron, Ohio call him "Tony." During these past two years, I would like to think that our friendship has grown because of the many conversations we've had. We've shared some really intimate and personal journey stories with each other. We've had many conversations where we've prayed for each other on the phone. It's really been great sharing with him and then him being able to capture my soul, my very essence in words. He is a phenomenal writer. The book will be published by fall of this year, and it will be dedicated to Fern... My Friend, My Big Sis, My Wisdom.

I will close by saying what I feel FERN meant to me, or should I say will always mean to me:

F is for Forever; I will forever be grateful for the times we shared, and I will never Forget you.

E is for the Everlasting friendship you've shown towards me.

R is for the Radiance that flows from you. AND FINALLY...

N is for that Nurturing Spirit that I will forever keep near my heart.

Rest in Peace. Big Sis. Rest in Peace.

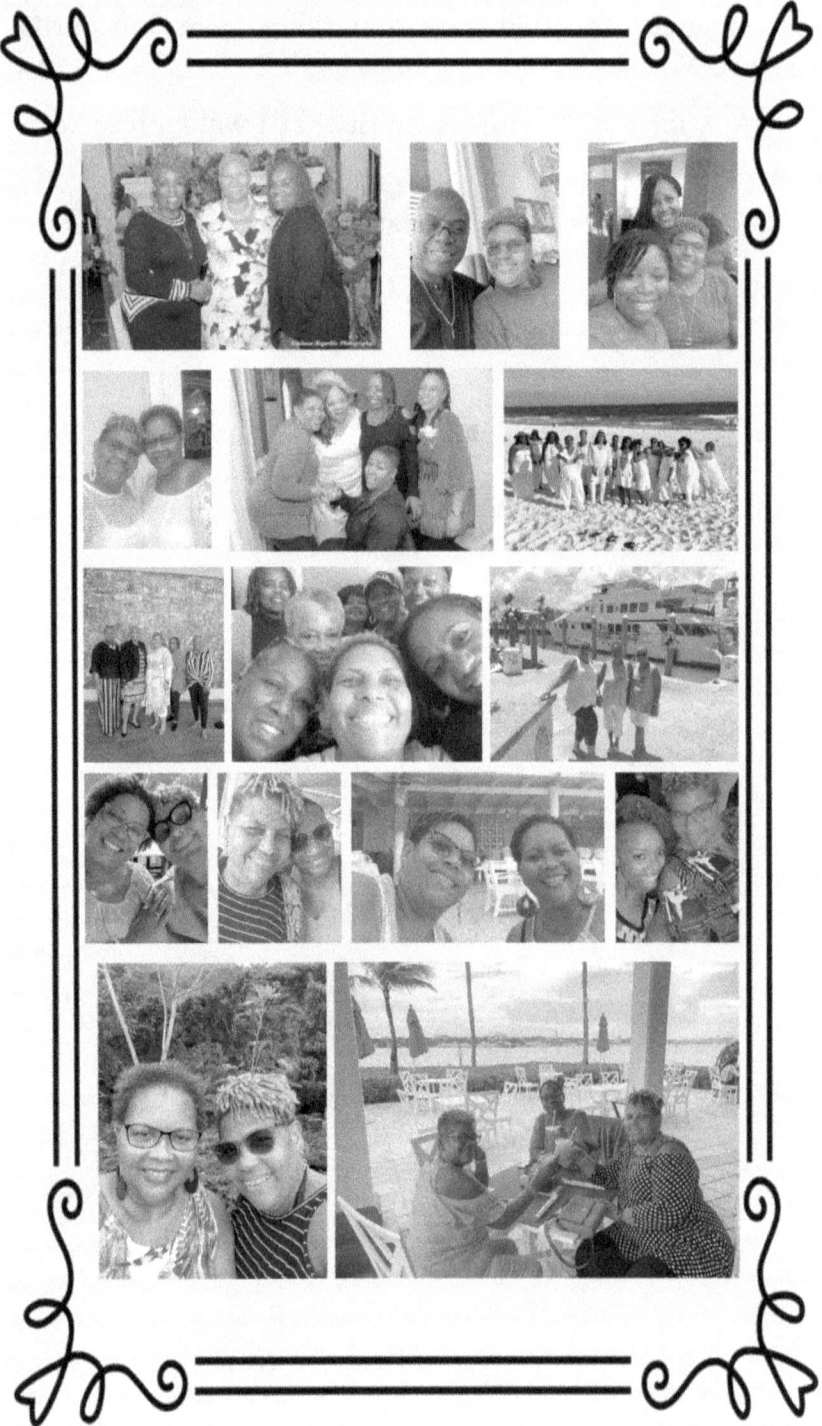

CHAPTER 10
A CLEAR SENSE OF LIFE
PURPOSE (GIVING BACK)

So, we've reached the final chapter in this book. As stated in the "Introduction," my ultimate goal in writing this book is to encourage and inspire other women who have gone through many of the same life experiences as I have. While being diagnosed with and struggling to survive breast cancer was a major obstacle I had to overcome, I didn't want to write a book that was solely focused on being a breast cancer survivor. I wanted to write a book that was about overcoming the limitations we place on ourselves, particularly as women. This includes allowing fear or the lack of courage to stop us from pursuing our greatest passions and vision for our life whether it is being an entrepreneur or letting go of an unhealthy and unfulfilling relationship.

This final chapter is entitled "A Clear Sense of Life Purpose" because the publishing of this book goes hand-in-hand with what I feel is a calling or sense of purpose for my life. That is, to inspire, empower and educate women on how to become healthy and whole persons and how to develop inner strength and courage to pursue their dreams and visions. A key aspect of fulfilling my life purpose is to actively coordinate and organize women— young and old—to have more formal and more meaningful conversations about the most pertinent aspects of our lives (e.g. What it means to be a mother? What it means to be a wife? How to forgive ourselves for our past failures in relationships with men and life in general? How to find balance in our personal lives while pursuing our career and professional goals?).

These are really tough questions to answer, frequently requiring us to wrestle with them before the right answer becomes crystal clear. In my estimation, compared to twenty, thirty years ago, fewer women are willing to wrestle with or even ask these critical questions. And, I believe this is a direct result of fewer women challenging one another as sisters, as friends and as peers. We need to hold each other accountable for the choices we make and the expectations we place on ourselves and those around us.

Woman 2 Woman is a literal and metaphorical concept that I developed and want to spread the word about throughout the United States and abroad. Metaphorically, it symbolizes the interconnectedness of women no matter their race, age or socioeconomic status. Literally, it is the inspiring of a movement of women who commit themselves to consistently and ritually sitting down to have face-to-face heart-to-heart conversations (*Woman 2 Woman*).

Ironically, as we were in the process of editing this book, the entire world was hit with the COVID-19 pandemic. In emphasizing the need for women to have more heart-to-heart conversations, this crisis reminded us of the incredible power of social media and modern technology. From the comfort of our own homes, we can communicate with anyone in the world. So, even if time does not permit you to meet in person, you have the luxury of using online technology platforms for face-to-face engagement.

This can occur in the kitchen of your home or apartment, at your church, in a gymnasium, a community center or even at your local library. The main thing is that we need to start talking to one another. Not just gossiping or engaging in surface level chatting. We need to start going below the surface. We need to have a willingness to look deeper, to dig deeper. We need to share more of the wisdom we've gained from our life experiences with one another. And, this will occur more frequently and more naturally when we begin to embrace and commit to the concept of "*Woman 2 Woman.*"

Before closing, I have to mention another major accomplishment and that is joining the sorority Delta Sigma Theta Sorority, Inc. Though I didn't join until I was age 50, I am a dues paying involved member for more than ten years. I have to give a shout out to my line sisters of "Hearts of Fire Rated R.E.D.D."

In addition, in this final chapter, I also would like to re-emphasize several key lessons, messages and themes that have been shared throughout this book in telling you my life story. I began by telling you how blessed I was to marry my childhood sweetheart and the amazing joy I have in raising two phenomenal sons. They are loving fathers, devoted husbands, college educated and just overall God-fearing, kind-hearted and I have to say, "GOOD-LOOKING" men. I, then, shared the courage it took for me to step out on faith with my business partner, of nearly thirty years, to start a business when we had very little money.

Forgiveness

Then, even though experiencing the excruciating pain of going through divorce, and not fully understanding how and why I lost a relationship that I thought would always be there, I had to find a way to move past the embarrassment, humiliation, hurt and pain. Amazingly, the answer that was revealed to me was totally unexpected. It was that I needed to focus my attention on "forgiveness" rather than feeling as though I was a victim. I needed to find something to give and share with others that was positive.

166

Equally important, I needed to be more aware of the words I spoke about my divorce. I needed to stop saying, "He left me." Rather, I needed to say "God has something even better for me. I just have to be willing to let go and open myself up to new blessings that WILL come into my life." And, that's exactly what happened when God sent Pete to me.

God has also opened so many other doors in my life because I committed myself to working on forgiveness. And, I am confident that these doors will not only continue to open but will open even wider now that my life purpose is clearer.

While encouraging women to have heart-to-heart conversations is central to fulfilling my life purpose, I cannot end this book without once again stressing the importance of early detection. God has given me a platform to share my story and to urge other women to get their mammograms. I am on a mission to get more women to understand the vital importance of getting a yearly mammogram and performing a monthly self-examination. Early detection is the key! If my breast cancer was not detected early, I would not have lived to tell my story. So, please, if you're over the age of 40 or have a family history of breast cancer, please schedule a mammogram as soon as possible!!!

Final Lessons/Thoughts

1. You've gotta keep it "movin!" Even when life throws you a curve ball, duck and keep moving.

2. "Don't give up" even though it sounds like a cliché'. DON'T EVER GIVE UP!

3. Keep a POSITIVE ATTITUDE when facing adversity in your life.

4. Find a Support Group. You would be surprised the number of people who are right where you are. Countless individuals are going through some of the very same things you're facing.

5. Be willing to encourage, support and walk with other women through their journey of facing and overcoming adversity in their lives.

6. Everyone has a story to tell. Isn't it time to tell YOURS!

7. God has a purpose for your life. Romans 9:17 ESV – *For the scriptures says to Pharaoh, "For this very purpose I have raised you up, that I might show my power in you. And that my name might be proclaimed in all the earth."*

8. Finally, remember these three things that I know to be true: God will never leave you. God never fails. And, God has a purpose for your life.

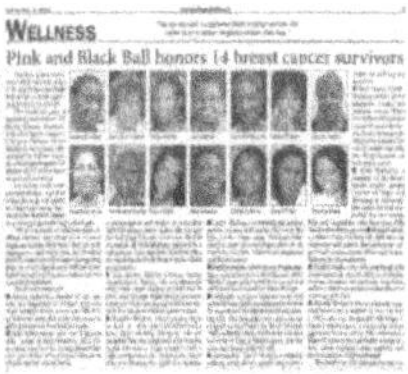

WELLNESS

Pink and Black Ball honors 14 breast cancer survivors

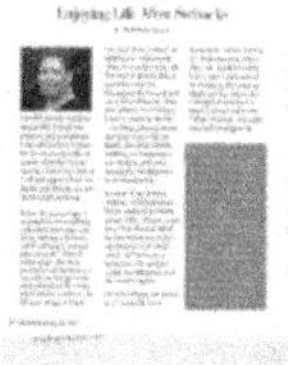

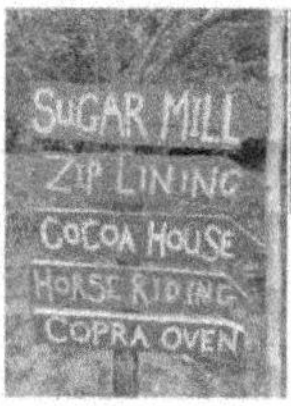

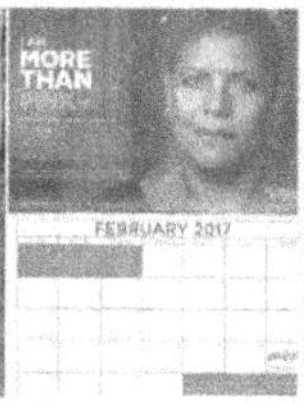

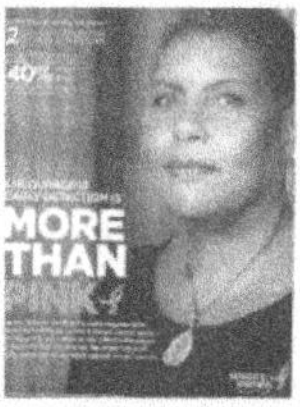

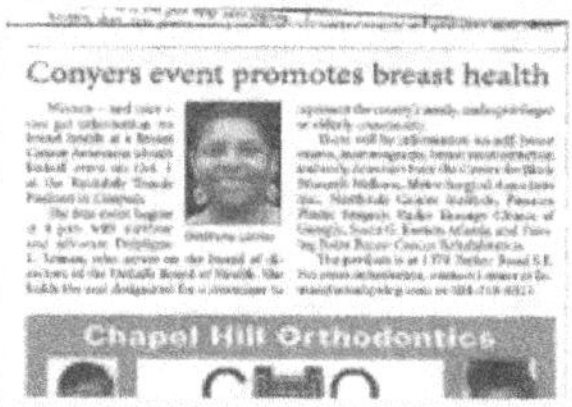

Conyers event promotes breast health

Chapel Hill Orthodontics

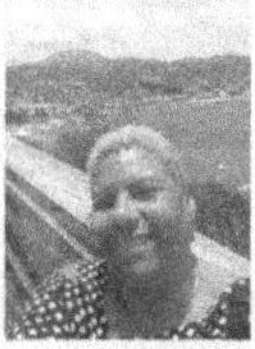

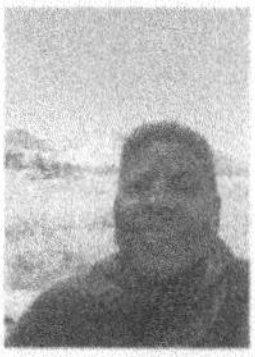

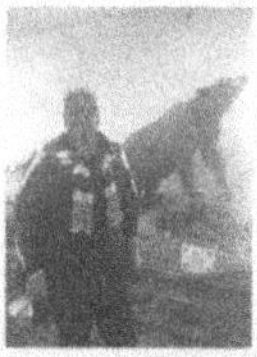

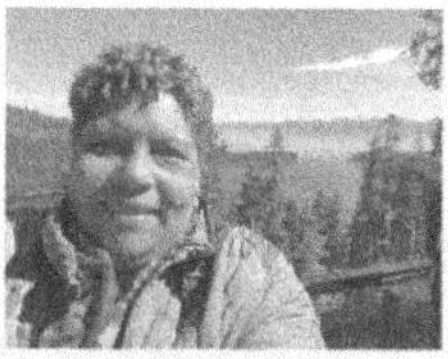

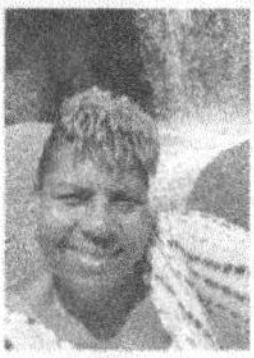

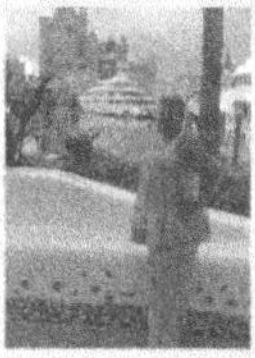

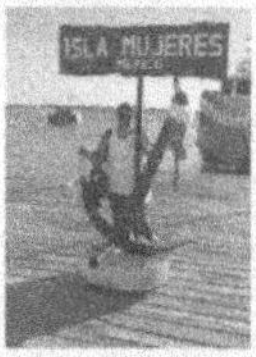

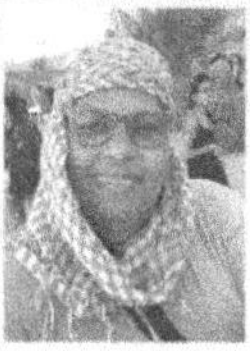

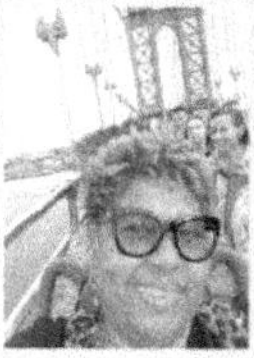

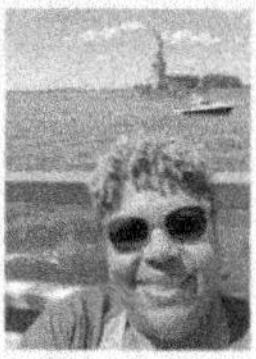

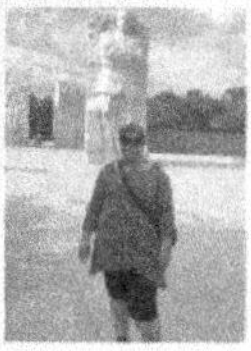

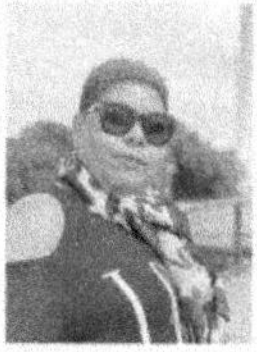

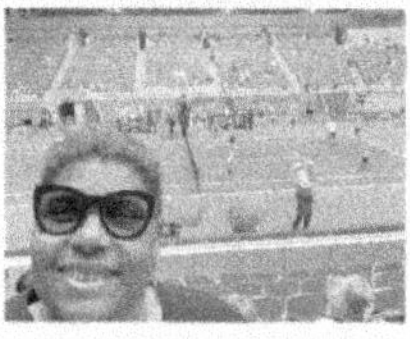

JOIN the *Woman 2 Woman* Movement!!!

Visit www.Woman2Woman.Network

- ❖ Sister's Circle (Support Groups)
- ❖ Gathering of The Sistah's
- ❖ Live Chats
- ❖ *Woman 2 Woman* Retreats
- ❖ Books
- ❖ Webinars
- ❖ Other Resources

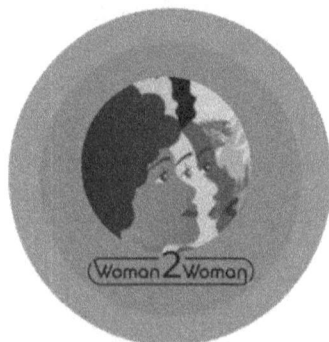

APPENDIX

For more information about breast cancer, you can also visit the website of the Susan G. Komen Breast Cancer Foundation:

https://ww5.komen.org/BreastCancer/BreastCancerScreeningforWomenatAverageRisk.html

https://ww5.komen.org/BreastCancer/BreastCancerScreeningForWomenAtHigherRisk.html

Figure 3.1 (below) shows the breast cancer screening recommend-dations for women at average risk from 3 major health organizations.

Learn about screening recommendations for women at higher than average risk of breast cancer.

Figure 3.1: Breast cancer screening recommendations for women at average risk		
American Cancer Society	**National Comprehensive Cancer Network**	**U.S. Preventive Services Task Force**
Mammography		
Informed decision-making with a health care provider age 40-44 Every year starting at age 45-54 Every 2 years (or every year if a woman chooses to do so) starting at age 55, for as long as a woman is in good health	Every year starting at age 40, for as long as a woman is in good health*	Informed decision-making with a health care provider age 40-49 Every 2 years ages 50-74

Clinical Breast Exam		
Not recommended	Every 1-3 years ages 25-39 Every year starting at age 40	Not enough evidence to recommend for or against
* 3D mammography (breast tomosynthesis) may be considered.		

Triple-Negative Breast Cancer

Triple-negative breast cancer is cancer that tests negative for estrogen receptors, progesterone receptors, and excess HER2 protein.

These results mean the growth of the cancer is not fueled by the hormones estrogen and progesterone, or by the HER2 protein. So, triple-negative breast cancer does not respond to hormonal therapy medicines or medicines that target HER2 protein receptors. Still, other medicines are used to successfully treat triple-negative breast cancer.

About 10-20% of breast cancers are triple-negative breast cancers. For doctors and researchers, there is intense interest in finding new medications that can treat this kind of breast cancer. Studies are trying to find out whether certain medications can interfere with the processes that cause triple-negative breast cancer to grow.

Three common features of triple-negative breast cancer

- **Triple-negative breast cancer is considered to be more aggressive and have a poorer prognosis than other types of breast cancer,** mainly because there are fewer targeted medicines that treat triple-negative breast cancer. Studies have shown that triple-negative breast cancer is more likely to spread beyond the breast and more likely to recur (come back) after treatment.

- **It tends to be higher grade than other types of breast cancer.** The higher the grade, the less the cancer cells resemble normal, healthy breast cells in their appearance and growth patterns. On a scale of 1 to 3, triple-negative breast cancer often is grade 3.

- **It usually is a cell type called "basal-like."** "Basal-like" means that the cells resemble the basal cells that line the breast ducts. Basal-like cancers tend to be more aggressive, higher grade cancers — just like triple-negative breast cancers. Most but not all basal-like breast cancers are triple negative, and most but not all triple-negative breast cancers are basal-like.

Who gets triple-negative breast cancer?

Anyone can be diagnosed with triple-negative breast cancer. Still, researchers have found that it is more common in:

- **Younger people.** Triple-negative breast cancer is more likely to be diagnosed in people younger than age 50. Other types of breast cancer are more commonly diagnosed in people age 60 or older.

- **African-American and Hispanic women.** Triple-negative breast cancer is more likely to be diagnosed in African-American women and Hispanic women. Asian women and non-Hispanic white women are less likely to be diagnosed with this type of cancer.

- **People with a BRCA1 mutation.** About 70% of breast cancers diagnosed in people with an inherited BRCA mutation, particularly BRCA1, are triple-negative

Source: BreastCancer.org

https://www.breastcancer.org/symptoms/diagnosis/trip_neg

https://simulations.kognito.com/tnbc/

NOTE: The statistics and references to research on breast cancer, listed above and throughout this book, were recorded on October 5, 2020 when this book was first published. Given the constant advances in research and treatment of cancer, new and more recent research and statistics will continually become available after the publication of this book.

Woman 2 Woman

www.ingramcontent.com/pod-product-compliance
Lightning Source LLC
Chambersburg PA
CBHW031300090426
42742CB00007B/533